EATING TO TREAT

GOUT

&

INFLAMMATION

200 RECIPES
FOR FOOD
THAT WILL
RELIEVE PAIN
& REDUCE
INFLAMMATION

Contents

INTRODUCTION

There is growing consensus among medical professionals that inflammation plays a major part in many of the chronic diseases that are fast becoming a plague of the Western World. All of these are on the increase. Irrespective of whether inflammation is the cause of these diseases or a result of them there is no doubt that inflammation provides a common link. While many are content to treat these chronic diseases with drugs, more and more doctors and physicians are beginning to accept that treating the underlying causes of the inflammation would be a better and more effective long term solution.

Gout has afflicted mankind for thousands of years. It is one of the most painful and debilitating diseases and it affects millions of people around the world. Today it is the most common form of inflammatory arthritis found in industrialised countries. In what is loosely described as the 'Western World' between 1% and 2% of men in their 50's and up to 7% of men in their 70's now suffer from gout. In the United States alone more than 6 million people suffer from gout. While hither too it was mainly a male disease women, particularly post menopausal women, are now being increasingly afflicted.

Why is gout increasing so rapidly? Possible explanations include lifestyle, high levels of pollution, the overall ageing of the population and the changes to our diet that have been made possible by increased prosperity and new food manufacturing processes.

If you have ever asked the question *"Why do I have gout"?* you will almost invariably have been told that it is because you have too much uric acid, something which is bound to be your fault as it is caused by eating too much purine rich food and drinking too much alcohol. The solution, drugs to reduce the amount of uric acid and a low purine diet. Notwithstanding that a rigid purine restricted diet is well nigh impossible to sustain for long, it is certainly not a diet that the rest of the family would enjoy eating. Ironically it is also a diet that is high in the foods that fuel inflammation and sadly lacking in the foods that calm it down.

When it comes to gout and inflammation you really are what you eat. Unfortunately the foods that can cause gout and inflammation are many, and they are foods that most of us in the west eat every day of our lives. The explanation of what these are and why they cause gout are the subject of another book, Goodbye To Gout - A New Gout Diet. For those of you who have not read this book some background information on inflammation is an essential first step to understanding how you can eat to treat gout and inflammation.

If you suffer from gout or another inflammatory disease one thing is certain, your whole body is in a state of inflammation and reducing that inflammation by eating less pro-inflammatory food and more anti inflammatory food is one of the most important things you can do. Not only will it take you to a different place physically and emotionally, it will also set you on the road to living an active gout and inflammation free life.

PART ONE

INFLAMMATION & OUR IMMUNE SYSTEM

Inflammation is a topic that is attracting a lot of attention at the moment. Gout is a form of inflammatory arthritis. When you are in the midst of a gout flare, the inflammation is all too obvious; redness, swelling and acute pain. But even when the gout flare has subsided the inflammation is still there, lurking in the wings and causing unseen damage. Because of this, understanding inflammation and how it affects your body is the essential first step on your road to recovery.

What Is Inflammation?

The word inflammation comes from the Latin word 'inflammo' meaning 'I set alight, I ignite'. When something harmful or irritating affects a part of your body there is an automatic response to try to remove it. When you catch a cold or sprain your ankle your immune system moves into gear and triggers a chain of events that is referred to as the inflammatory cascade. The familiar signs of inflammation, raised temperature, localised heat, pain, swelling and redness, are the first signs that your immune system is being called into action and they show you that your body is trying to heal itself.

Innate & Adaptive Immunity

Inflammation is part of the body's 'innate' immune response, something that is present even before we are born. Innate immunity is an automatic immunity that is not directed towards anything specific. As we go through life and are exposed to diseases or vaccinated against them we acquire 'adaptive' immunity. In a delicate balance of give-and-take inflammation begins when 'pro-inflammatory hormones' in your body call out for your white blood cells to come and clear out an infection or repair damaged tissue. These pro-inflammatory hormones are matched by equally powerful closely related 'anti-inflammatory' compounds which move in once the threat is neutralised to begin the healing process.

Acute & Chronic Inflammation

The inflammation we experience during our daily lives can be either 'acute' or 'chronic'. Chronic inflammation is sometimes referred to as 'systemic' inflammation.

Acute inflammation that ebbs and flows as needed signifies a well balanced immune system. Colds, flu and childhood diseases mean that inflammation and a rise in temperature starts suddenly and quickly progresses to become severe. The signs and symptoms are only present for a few days and they soon subside. On occasion, in cases of severe illness, they can sometimes last for a few weeks but this is unusual.

Sometimes, however, as in the case of chronic or systemic inflammation, the inflammation itself can cause further inflammation. It can become self perpetuating and sometimes last for months or even years. Symptoms of inflammation that do not go away are telling you that the switch to your immune system is stuck in the 'on' position. It is poised on high alert and is unable to shut itself off. Some people believe that chronic irritants, food sensitivities and common allergens like the proteins found in dairy products and wheat can trigger this type of chronic inflammation.

The Link Between Gout & Your Immune System

The study of inflammation and our immune system is a relatively new science. While there is still an enormous amount to learn there is no doubt that the human immune response is an extremely sophisticated finely balanced mechanism. Without it we would not be able to survive the most minor infection or the tiniest cut. Some scientists believe that like other things in our evolutionary history, this sophisticated immune response gave our early ancestors a major survival advantage. As with so much about the human body, how such a sophisticated response came about is unclear. It is certainly the subject of a great deal of speculation.

If you suffer from gout you will almost certainly have heard of uric acid, mainly because it is regarded as being the 'bad guy'. Man and our ancestors, the higher primates, are the only mammals that have uric acid and some scientists believe that evolution may have had a major incentive in giving us uric acid.

Inflammation occurs when tissues in our body are damaged or when we are 'attacked' by bacteria or viruses. Substances like pro inflammatory hormones are produced by our body and these alert it to the danger and tell our immune system to switch itself on. Uric acid behaves like one of these pro inflammatory hormones. It is not involved in our immune response to bacteria and viruses but it is involved when our bodies are subjected to trauma and when our cells are damaged or die. The large amounts of uric acid that are produced in the immediate vicinity of damaged, dying or dead cells stimulate a type of immune cell called dendritic cells to mature and swing into action. Effectively uric acid has a sort of 'immune boosting' effect and it plays a fundamental part in protecting our bodies from tissue damage and trauma. If this theory is correct, uric acid came to the rescue of the higher primates and enabled them to develop an extremely robust defence against injury and large scale tissue damage. Without doubt, this would have given them a substantial survival advantage.

Inflammatory Markers & Chemical Messengers

In the Western World chronic or systemic inflammation is on the rise. We know this from inflammatory markers and the pro inflammatory and anti inflammatory hormones that our body's produce. One of the inflammatory markers, C-Reactive Protein, (CRP) is a protein that binds to bacteria and dead and dying cells in order to clear them out from our body. CRP can always be found and measured in our blood stream, but levels of CRP spike when there is inflammation. CRP is highly sensitive and its' levels increase rapidly in response to any type of inflammation. CRP tells us that inflammation is present but it doesn't tell us what is causing the inflammation.

Interleukin-6 (IL-6) is another inflammatory maker that is secreted by two different types of cells; white blood cells called T-cells, and another type of cell called macrophages. The macrophages are the cells that engulf and digest stray tissue and pathogens. T-cells and macrophages play a huge role in our immune response.

Chronic or systemic inflammation does not result in the sweeping response of trauma but it does keep the body in a constant state of being 'in repair' mode. Immune cells like the macrophages take charge and a recurring process of tissue destruction and repair takes over.

The Chemical Messengers Within Our Cells

Without getting into the biochemistry in too much detail, there is a complicated interaction between the inflammatory chemical messengers that are inside our bodies; cytokines, prostaglandins and the short lived hormones inside our cells called eicosanoids. Understanding these is key to understanding a major element of how we can eat to treat gout and inflammation.

Eicosanoids

These are interesting as they can act as both pro-inflammatory compounds that can 'fuel' inflammation and anti-inflammatory compounds that can calm it down. Put simply, the anti-inflammatory eicosanoids draw upon one group of compounds in our tissues and the pro-inflammatory eicosanoids on another set of compounds. In order to maintain a proper inflammatory response we need both of these eicosanoids in a relative state of balance. However with high levels of the compounds the pro-inflammatory eicosanoids need and low levels of the compounds the anti-inflammatory compounds need we end up making far too many pro-inflammatory eicosanoids and not enough of the anti-inflammatory ones.

Cytokines

These are a group of proteins that are secreted by specific cells in our immune system. Each different cytokine has a specific function. Cytokines act as chemical messengers between our cells, managing and regulating various inflammatory responses such as immunity and inflammation.

Prostaglandins

These are another type of chemical messenger that our bodies use, but first a little about enzymes.

An enzyme is a substance that enables a chemical reaction to take place, they act as a 'catalyst'. The chemical reaction can not take place unless the enzyme is present. However, in the process of helping with the chemical reaction the enzyme itself is not changed, it acts as a sort of facilitator. Enzymes are able to catalyse tens of thousands of reactions at the same time. They are extremely efficient. Our bodies contain thousands of different enzymes and each of these is finely tuned to undertake a specific task.

The prostaglandins mentioned earlier are made from specific compounds in our body by two different enzymes that are called COX-1 and COX-2. The prostaglandins in our bodies have slightly different effects that are dependent on which of these COX-1 and COX-2 enzymes were used when they were made. The COX-1 enzyme is always present but the COX-2 enzyme is not usually detectable in normal tissue, it only becomes abundant at the sites of inflammation. If you suffer from gout you will have heard of NSAID's, Non Steroidal Anti-inflammatory Drugs. These work by blocking the COX-1 and COX-2 enzymes and preventing them from forming the inflammatory prostaglandins.

Stress, Lifestyle & Inflammation

Does lifestyle play a part in inflammation? In a word yes, and the impact of lifestyle can be greater than you think.

Believe it or not stress can be a killer. Our body is hard wired to protect us from the threat of danger. If you have ever had a panic attack or woken from a really frightening dream in a cold sweat with your heart pounding you will understand only too well what acute stress feels like.

All human beings have a natural alarm system of *'fight or flight'* so when we are angry, anxious, tense and generally on edge our bodies produce a surge of hormones that prepare us for the fight that lies ahead. They increase our heart rate, increase our blood pressure and give rise to a sudden boost of energy. Cortisol, the primary stress hormone, increases the amount of glucose in our blood stream and enhances the way our brain and body uses this glucose. In anticipation of any damage that is likely to occur it also alters our immune system and puts our body's inflammatory response onto high alert. The poor sleep quality and short sleep duration that comes with stress also leads to increased levels of inflammatory markers.

Simply having gout makes you feel stressed, not least because of the pain, the constant 'why me?' the dread of the next attack and the utter hopelessness of the situation you find yourself in. Breaking the stress cycle is no easy task.

The body's stress response system is usually self regulating but when stress in life is always present our body is over exposed to Cortisol and other stress hormones and these then begin to disrupt many of our body's processes, creating a state of chronic inflammation that weakens our immune system and interferes with proper glucose metabolism and the release of insulin. Ultimately this leads to insulin resistance and a general state of oxidative stress, all of which has the effect of increasing levels of uric acid and inflammation.

What Happens When You Have a Gout Flare?

Gout flares are caused by uric acid that has formed crystals. Often these crystals lodge in the connective tissue in a joint, the big toe being a common place. How and why these crystals develop is explained in Goodbye To Gout: A New Gout Diet. However, once crystals have formed the first gout attack will almost inevitably follow. When this happens the body's innate immune response quickly detects the newly appearing uric acid crystals and assumes that they are diseased or damaged cells. In response, white blood cells are sent to attack the 'invaders', but when they try to devour them the uric acid crystals burst the white blood cells. As the white blood cells die, they release proteins telling the immune system that they have lost their fight with the invader and that reinforcements need to be sent in. The released proteins also generate something called lactic acid and this makes the blood slightly more acidic than it should be.

In order to bring the acidity of the blood back to normal something called our *phosphate buffering system* swings into action. When this happens minute particles of calcium are sometimes released and this causes more crystals of uric acid to form around the tiny particles of calcium. The immune system responds by sending in more white blood cells. More white blood cells are killed by the uric acid crystals causing even more proteins and lactic acid to be released and more crystals to form. This process perpetuates itself, creating a runaway inflammatory response and the extreme pain of gout.

Ultimately the process is self limiting because the concentration of uric acid reduces as it is consumed by the growing crystals and gradually the acidity of the blood returns to normal. This explains the fact that uric acid levels often reduce during a gout attack, sometimes to within normal ranges. However, after the gout flare has subsided you are left with what is effectively a permanent low grade systemic inflammation with increased levels of C- Reactive Protein and inflammatory cytokines and a body that in immunological terms is 'sensitised' and in a state of high alert, waiting for the next attack.

PART TWO

THE BUILDING BLOCKS OF OUR IMMUNE SYSTEM

The human body is a complex organism. It is a massive biological engine that is fuelled by the food we eat and the air we breathe. In the cells that make up our bodies thousands of different biochemical reactions are taking place each second, converting food and oxygen into the energy we need and the compounds that make up our bodies. Together these complex chemical reactions make up our metabolism.

The Building Blocks

Food is consumed, broken down and transformed into the enormous number of different compounds and materials that our body needs and not least among these are the enzymes, hormones and prostaglandins that make up our immune system.

In order to understand inflammation, our immune system and the way in which we can eat to treat gout and inflammation, we need to understand the role that the different types of food we eat plays in our body. Key to this are proteins, carbohydrates and fats. Of these three, carbohydrates and fats are the most important when it comes to inflammation but free radicals and anti-oxidants also play a critical role.

Free Radicals & Antioxidants.

Free Radicals

The majority of life forms that exist on earth need oxygen to live, yet one of the paradoxes of this is that oxygen is a highly reactive molecule that can damage living organisms by producing Free Radicals. These are compounds, atoms or molecules that are highly unstable because of their structure. Any molecule or atom that has one or more unpaired or 'free' electrons in its outer orbit is known as a free radical. Free radicals attempt to make themselves stable by reacting with other atoms and molecules. In order to do this they either 'steal' an electron from them, bind to another molecule or interact in various ways with other free radicals. This is a process that is referred to as oxidation.

Simply by living and deriving energy from the air we breathe and the food we eat our bodies produce free radicals. Many of these are needed in controlled amounts to maintain life and keep us in good health. Our immune systems depends heavily on them. Others however can cause damage, sometimes severe damage, by reacting with cells, fats and proteins inside our bodies. Free radicals are all around us. We breath them in from cigarette smoke, car exhausts and air pollution, the ultra violet rays from the sun create them when we are exposed to sunlight and we consume them in our food and often in the water we drink.

An imbalance or overload of free radicals can impair our immune system and it is a potential factor in many modern day illnesses. In order for us to be able to lead healthy lives the Free Radicals need to be neutralised and rendered harmless and to do this we need antioxidants.

Antioxidants

The word antioxidants refers to any molecule that is capable of deactivating free radicals and making them stable. Unlike free radicals which have electrons missing, antioxidants are molecules that have electrons to spare. When antioxidants come into contact with free radicals they hand over their spare electrons and neutralise the free radicals by binding to them and effectively 'making them safe'. The human body has a highly complex internally produced defence against free radicals, a sophisticated armoury of antioxidants that is uses to defend and protect itself by inhibiting the formation of free radicals, neutralising free radicals that are already formed and repairing any damage that free radicals have caused. In addition to our bodies own antioxidant defence team, antioxidants are contained in the food we eat; Vitamin C, Vitamin E and the beta carotenes are just some of the 8,000 antioxidants that nature provides us with in our food.

For many years uric acid was considered to be an inert waste product that, when present in higher than normal levels, was known for the harmful and troublesome effects of causing gout and kidney stones. Even now many sources of information on gout tell you that "uric acid serves no biochemical function". Well, we now know much more about uric acid's various biochemical functions and one of these is that it is a powerful antioxidant. In fact uric acid has the highest concentration of any of the water soluble antioxidants found in our blood and it provides nearly half of the antioxidant capacity that our blood contains. Its antioxidant properties are fifty times as powerful as those of Vitamin C.

When our antioxidant defences are over powered by free radicals and when free radicals increase at a rate that is faster than our body's ability to increase its own antioxidant defences, the disturbance in the antioxidant to pro-oxidant balance shifts in favour of the free radicals and damage to the body and Oxidative Stress develops.

Oxidative Stress

Oxidative Stress exists when there is an imbalance between free radicals and the body's ability to render them harmless or repair the damage they have caused. The body either has an inadequate supply of antioxidants or it is creating or being exposed to too many free radicals. When this happens the free radicals oxidise and damage cells and other components of the cells. This leads to the influx of inflammatory cells at the sites of the injury and inevitably an increase in uric acid.

The effect of Oxidative Stress depends on the size or scale of the imbalance between the free radicals and the antioxidants. A cell is able to overcome small amounts of damage and regain its original state, but more severe Oxidative Stress can have toxic effects that can on occasion result in widespread cell death. Whatever happens, the result is inflammation and the severity of this inflammation will correspond to the scale of the Oxidative Stress and the level of imbalance between the free radicals and antioxidants.

Proteins & Amino Acids

Proteins are the main tissue builders in our body. They exist in every cell and they are essential for all of the body's functions. Many proteins are the enzymes that act as the catalysts for the biochemical reactions that take place when we breakdown and metabolise the food we eat. They also play an important part in our body's immune response.

Proteins are made from amino acids. These are organic compounds that are mainly, but not exclusively, made from the elements carbon, hydrogen, oxygen and nitrogen. About 500 different amino acids are known and they are classified into different groups. In the form of proteins they comprise the second largest component after water in human muscles, cells and tissues.

Carbohydrates

Carbohydrates are the most abundant biological molecules and they fulfil numerous roles in our bodies. They are produced by most green plants as an energy store. The food we eat supplies us with carbohydrates in two different forms, starch and sugar. Both of these also contain fibre or cellulose. Starches and sugars provide us with energy. Fibre or cellulose provides us with the 'bulk' our digestive systems need to work efficiently.

In technical terms all carbohydrates, including the fibre and cellulose they contain, are sugars. They consist of single, double or multiple units of sugar that are joined together in different ways. Simple sugars are only one or two units long and they are typically sweet in taste whereas complex carbohydrates can be thousands of sugar units long and they have a starchy taste.

With the exception of a sugar called fructose all carbohydrates, irrespective of whether they are starch or sugar, are digested or metabolised by our body to form glucose, a simple form of sugar that our body uses as a source of fuel to generate energy.

Fibre and Cellulose

Carbohydrates contain two types of fibre, soluble fibre and insoluble fibre. Insoluble fibre is a non digestible complex carbohydrate. It does not dissolve in water and is not fermented by the bacteria in our digestive system because we do not possess the enzymes needed to break the links between the sugar units apart.

Soluble fibre does dissolve in water and it is fermented by the bacteria and micro organisms in our large intestine.

Starchy Carbohydrates

Starchy carbohydrates contain two types of starch. One of these is a high glycemic starch that is absorbed and converted into glucose very easily and surprisingly quickly. This gives you a fast 'glucose hit' and any glucose that is not needed as an immediate energy source is stored in various buffer stores around our body. When these buffer stores become full the excess glucose ultimately finds its way to our fat cells.

The other starchy carbohydrate is known as Resistant Starch and it is called resistant starch simply because it is much more difficult for our bodies to digest it. It takes longer to digest and the starch in it is released much more slowly. Because of this some people regard resistant starch as a third type of fibre as it provides the benefits of both soluble and insoluble fibre.

Resistant starch has attracted quite a lot of attention over recent years. Many studies have shown that it is a natural appetite suppressant because it is able to turn on some enzymes that boost the hormones that make you feel full and stay full for longer. Several studies have also shown that it helps people burn fat and increase their insulin sensitivity. Because our diets are high in refined carbohydrates, most people consume far too little resistant starch, something in the order of 5 grams a day. Researchers believe that we should be consuming twice if not three times this amount.

Sugar

A carbohydrate that we have all heard of and it is quite rightly receiving a really bad press. So what exactly is sugar? First and foremost sugar is a natural food. It only becomes unnatural when it is in a form, concentration or quality that is not found in nature, High Fructose Corn Syrup is an example of this. Sugar comes in several forms and many disguises. The most common form is sucrose or what we know as table sugar. This is a 'dissacharide', a compound that is made up of one molecule of glucose that is linked to one molecule of fructose. So it contains 50% glucose and 50% fructose. When our bodies metabolise sugar it is converted into separate molecules of glucose and fructose. Each of these are simple sugars or 'monosaccharides'. There is a third monosaccharide called galactose. All other types of sugar are made from combinations of these three monosaccharides, glucose, fructose and galactose.

Glucose is the most important sugar as it is provides the primary source of fuel that is used throughout our body. Our body stores glucose in the liver and in our muscles in the form of glycogen and this can be easily and quickly broken down back into glucose to provide energy when we need it.

Galactose is the least common simple monosaccharide sugar. It is found mainly in dairy products in the form of lactose, which is one molecule of galactose linked to one molecule of glucose. In this form it is easily converted into glucose when it is metabolised.

Fructose is found in fruit. Unlike galactose it cannot be converted into glucose or used throughout our body. If our body is desperately short of glucose our muscles can use fructose but as this rarely happens when we are consuming a typical 'Western Diet' most of the fructose we consume is converted into glycogen by the liver. If the glycogen stores in the liver are full fructose is rapidly converted into fat.

Contrary to what we are often led to believe the fructose found in whole fruit is not 'bad' as such as the rate at which it is absorbed is slowed down by the fibre the fruit contains. However, the fructose found in fruit juice is most definitely 'bad' as we consume far more fructose in a glass of orange juice than we would if we were eating the whole oranges. The juice in a standard glass of orange juice is equivalent to the juice of three to four oranges. As almost all of the fibre in the oranges has been removed during the manufacturing process a large amount of fructose is absorbed very rapidly and quickly converted into fat when we drink orange juice or other fruit juices.

Fats (Lipids) & Fatty Acids

In terms of inflammation and our immune response fats and fatty acids are probably the most important group of foods that we need to understand.

Lipid is the medical term for fat. It is a term that is usually used to refer to the fats that are found in our blood. Lipids and fats are the most diverse group of biochemicals in our body. They are regarded as the third food group after carbohydrates and proteins. Lipids and fats are a class of organic compound that are sometimes referred to as 'Fatty Acids'.

There are three different groups of lipids in our body, Triglycerides, Phospholipids and Sterols, also known as Steroids. The Triglycerides are the commonest and the most relevant to inflammation.

Fats and Lipids are a class of organic substances that are not soluble in water. In simple terms they are made from chains of carbon and hydrogen atoms that are 'bound' together in different ways and held together at one end by a sort of "head' that is made from carbon and oxygen atoms. The chains come in different lengths, they are twisted together and 'bent' in different ways and they come with different degrees of 'saturation'.

A fat is 'saturated' when all of the available atoms of carbon and hydrogen are linked together and this makes them very stable. Because they are stable they do not react with oxygen and oxidise and produce free radicals, or in technical terms become 'rancid', even when they are heated for cooking purposes. As a general rule the more saturated a fat is the more stable it is and the more beneficial and safer it is to eat.

Triglycerides can be divided into three groups:-

Saturated fats:
These have no free atoms of hydrogen, do not oxidise and produce free radicals easily and are solid at room temperature.

Monounsaturated fats:
These have two hydrogen atoms missing and are usually liquid at room temperature. Like saturated fats they are relatively stable and do not oxidise or 'go rancid' easily.

Polyunsaturated fats:
These have four or more hydrogen atoms missing and are liquid even when cold. These fats are very unstable and highly reactive. Even in their natural state polyunsaturated fats oxidise and produce free radicals very easily and this is why nature has packaged them up inside nuts and seeds that are packed full of the antioxidants and vitamins needed to protect them from oxidation. As a consequence, once they are extracted from the nuts and seeds these oils become chemically highly reactive and are characterised by very high levels of free radicals. When polyunsaturated fats are heated for cooking purposes the amount of these free radicals increases at an alarming rate.

Polyunsaturated fats are referred to as PUFA's, Polyunsaturated Fatty Acids. They are found in different amounts in all natural foods including meat, fish, vegetables and seeds. In general, vegetable oils such as sunflower, safflower, corn, soy, flax seed, sesame seed, pumpkin seed and canola oils are the most concentrated sources of PUFA's in our diet. The problem with all of these is the amount of free radicals they contain and the load that these put on our body's antioxidant defences. But the storey does not end there. For years we have been told that butter is bad for us and that margarine is a healthier option. However, when margarine is made a process called 'hydrogenation' is used to convert polyunsaturated fats that are liquid at room temperature into Trans Fats that are solid at room temperature. In reality Trans Fats are Polyunsaturated Vegetable Oils (PUFA') in their worst possible form and they are found in just about all of the processed food we eat today.

The manufacturing process of Hydrogenation is far from being a healthy process and not surprisingly the end result of the process is not a healthy product. Polyunsaturated oils that are already heavy in free radicals from the extraction process are mixed with a catalyst that is then subjected to hydrogen gas in a high pressure, high temperature reactor. Hence 'hydrogenated'. Emulsifiers and starch are then added to improve the consistency and the oil is again subjected to high temperatures in order to steam clean it and remove any unpleasant smells. Bleach, dyes and flavours are then added to make it look like and taste like butter. By the time margarine reaches your table it is a completely unnatural product and hardly the healthy food it is promoted as being. Trans fats are polyunsaturated vegetable oils in their worst possible form with even more free radicals than the polyunsaturated vegetable oils they were derived from, and the bad news is that we are consuming them in alarming amounts.

Fatty acids contain different types of fats in different proportions. They are broadly classified into 4 groups; Omega-3, Omega-6, Omega-9 and Conjugated fatty acids. Each of these four groups contains a number of different types of fatty acids.

Essential Fatty Acids or EFA's

Most of us have heard about Essential Fatty Acids, the names Omega-3 and Omega-6 usually come to mind. But what exactly are they and why are they so important?

Our bodies are able to make most of the different types of fats and fatty acids that it needs from the food we eat. However, some of the fats we need can only be obtained directly from our food. Because our bodies are unable to make them these fats are called Essential Fatty Acids or EFA's. Without these fatty acids our body would not function. They provide fats to the brain and nerves, they are needed for the structural and functional parts of our cell membranes and they play a major role in supporting our immune system and our immune cells.

Alpha Linolenic Acid (ALA) and Linoleic Acid (LA) are the two Essential Fatty Acid's that are of most interest as they are the 'parents' so to speak of the different groups of Omega-3 and Omega-6 fatty acids that our bodies make from them.

Alpha Linolenic Acid (ALA) is the parent of the Omega-3 group of Essential Fatty Acids and it is converted by our body into eicosapentaenoic acid (EPA) and decosahexaenoic acid (DHA). Unfortunately this conversion process is not very efficient and some scientists believe that as little as 1% of the ALA we consume ends up as DHA or EPA. To make matters worse this 1% conversion process decreases even more as we get older. Luckily both DHA and EPA can be obtained directly from our food so we need to obtain a lot of DHA and EPA as well as ALA from our diet. Sadly the modern Western Diet does not provide a very good source of any of these Omega-3 fats.

Linoleic Acid (LA) is the parent of the Omega-6 group of Essential Fatty Acids and it is converted by our bodies into Gamma-Linolenic acid (GLA) and Arachidonic Acid (AA). Unlike ALA, Linoleic Acid it is readily converted into GLA and AA and our Western Diet provides an abundant source of Linoleic Acid.

As well as playing several crucial roles in our body the Omega-3 group of fatty acids, EPA and DHA, have powerful anti-inflammatory properties, not least because the anti-inflammatory group of *Eicosanoid compounds* mentioned earlier are derived from EPA, Eicosapentaenoic Acid

The Omega-6 fatty acids GLA and AA have powerful pro-inflammatory properties. The pro-inflammatory group of *Eicosanoid compounds* are derived from them. Our Western Diet, which is high in polyunsaturated vegetable oils, provides an abundant source of the Omega-6 parent, Linoleic Acid. This means that we end up with an imbalance in the ratio of Omega 3 and Omega 6 and this has a profound effect on gearing up the inflammation process. Put simply, our modern diet of vegetable oils and trans fats is taking its toll. We are making too many pro inflammatory compounds and not enough anti inflammatory ones. Add to this the increased load of free radicals that the vegetable oils and trans fats bring with them it is easy to see that our body and immune system is being put under enormous stress.

Our Digestive System

What has our digestive system got to do with inflammation?

Many doctor's believe that the seeds of chronic inflammation as well as a lot of other health issues start with our digestive system, simply because they estimate that two thirds of our body's immune defences reside in our gastrointestinal tract.

Our Gastrointestinal tract is designed to destroy the viruses and bacteria in our food before they infect our body, so it is hardly surprising that our immune system clicks rapidly into action in our digestive tract.

There are hundreds of different types of bacteria in our digestive tract and over the years scientists have discovered that the number and type of bacteria can have a profound effect on our health. Our stomach uses acid to kill disease causing microbes and other nasties but it allows beneficial microbes which are acid tolerant to pass through into our small intestine. If your stomach is unsuccessful at getting rid of the 'bad guys' they can make their way to the small intestine and dominate your digestive tract, damaging the walls of the intestine and making you ill. Interestingly, our stomach becomes less acidic as we get older, so as we age the number of beneficial microbes reduces.

When we consume what is ubiquitously called 'junk food', for various reasons which are discussed later, bad, unfriendly microbes begin to flourish and good, friendly microbes begin to decline. The bad microbes produce endotoxins which our immune system detects as invaders that must be removed. The normal immune response is switched on and the start of an inflammatory cascade begins.

Common allergens like the casein found in milk and the gluten found in wheat can also be quick to spark an inflammatory cascade but stress is also a well known disruptor of the the digestive system. If you have ever lost your appetite, felt sick or had bad diarrhoea before an exam or an important interview you will know what I mean.

There is evidence that stress inhibits the way your small intestine absorbs glucose, fructose and galactose. When this happens sugars end up making their way to the large intestine where they are fermented by the bacteria there and this can lead to discomfort and flatulence. More important though, is that stress has an immediate impact on both the composition and function of the bacteria in our digestive tract and this can make the population of bacteria less diverse. As a consequence the sort of bad bacteria that can cause damage begin to take over.

PART THREE

THE FOOD WE EAT & INFLAMMATION

It is clear that some foods are inflammatory because they promote and fuel inflammation, and that some foods are anti-inflammatory because they calm inflammation down. We've talked about Proteins, Carbohydrates and the Essential Fatty Acids so how does the food we eat during our day by day lives fit into the big picture of inflammation?

Understanding Inflammatory & Anti-Inflammatory Foods

How do we know which foods are inflammatory and which foods are anti-inflammatory?

 As a general rule carbohydrates and meat are inflammatory, all fish, vegetables and fruit, with only a few exceptions, are anti-inflammatory. What a food contains as well as the way it is cooked affects its inflammatory potential. For instance, a boiled potato is far less inflammatory than a fried or roasted one, especially when it is fried or roasted in vegetable oil. Onions that are eaten raw or lightly sautéed are highly anti-inflammatory but cover them in batter and fry them in vegetable oil and they become highly inflammatory.

The type and amount of fat and Essential Fatty Acids a food contains is a key element when determining its inflammatory potential, but the vitamins, minerals and antioxidants it contains, the amount and type of carbohydrate, fibre and resistant starch, as well as other nutrients and anti-inflammatory compounds like polyphenols, all combine to predict the effect the different types of food will have on our bodies. Various organisations have published 'Inflammation Factors', 'Inflammation Indexes' and 'Inflammation Ratings' using their own preparatory scoring systems, but with so many different factors coming into play it is not surprising that there is as yet no agreed 'standard' for measuring the inflammation potential of specific foods.

If you look on the internet you will find sites that publish lists of how inflammatory or anti-inflammatory different foods are, but because of the different ways in which these lists have been calculated, the figures vary quite considerably. They do however give a reasonable indication of a food's inflammatory potential.

Which are the most strongly anti-inflammatory foods and which are the most strongly pro-inflammatory foods?

Cold water oily fish like salmon, herring and mackerel are by far the most anti-inflammatory foods you can eat. In fact, without exception, all fish and seafood is anti-inflammatory, provided of course that it is not covered in batter or breadcrumbs and fried in vegetable oil. Surprisingly many herbs and spices like garlic, chilli, ginger, cinnamon and turmeric, even in small amounts, are strongly anti-inflammatory and onions, carrots, sweet potatoes, spinach, squashes and kale also come high on the list.

When it comes to the most inflammatory foods you won't be surprised to hear that it is meat and poultry, offal, sugar, refined carbohydrates, food that is fried in vegetable oil and processed foods that contain trans fats.

At first sight the classification of some foods can be very confusing, especially as some foods contain both both pro-inflammatory and anti-inflammatory compounds. An orange for example contains large amounts of antioxidants that help reduce inflammation, but it also contains quite a large amount of the sugar fructose which can fuel inflammation. Oatmeal is another example as, like all grains, it is generally classed as being moderately inflammatory. However, there are many people who regard oatmeal as a sort of 'superfood' because it has low levels of fat, it is high in protein, it contains little or no gluten and it has very high levels of resistant starch, something which is lacking in our modern diet. Oatmeal also contains a fibre called beta-glucan and a powerful anti-oxidant called avenanthramide and both of these have a beneficial effect on reducing levels of bad cholesterol.

At the end of the day it is all about balance. If you lived on nothing but oatmeal you would not have a very good diet, but if you combine a bowl of unsweetened porridge with a chopped apple, a handful of cherries or some lightly sautéed vegetables you immediately balance out the 'inflammatory' potential of the oatmeal and give yourself a very healthy meal.

Do our bodies reflect our foods' inflammation potential?

The answer to this is interesting as several 'day-by-day' and 'diary' dietary studies have shown that they do but not to the extent that you would expect. However, when you look at large epidemiological studies the picture is completely different.

Inflammation is a bit like an iceberg floating on the sea. The top, like the visible signs of inflammation, is clear to see, but under the surface there is an awful lot of ice, completely hidden from view. Chronic and systemic inflammation is like the ice below the surface. The chemical 'markers', CRP and Interleukin-6 in our bodies indicate how inflamed our bodies are. By measuring these markers across large populations it is clear that those of us who consume the standard 'Western Diet' have much higher levels of these inflammatory markers than populations that consume a 'Mediterranean Diet'.

When you look at the typical 'Western Diet' it is easy to see that it contains large amounts of red and processed meat, high fat dairy products, over refined carbohydrates, sugar, vegetable oils and trans fats. It is low in fish, very low in fresh vegetables and fruit and sadly lacking in fibre and resistant starch. On the other hand the Mediterranean Diet is the opposite. It contains large amounts of fresh vegetables and fruit, fish and fibre. It contains moderate amounts of olive oil, which incidentally is anti-inflammatory, and red wine. It is low in red meat, processed foods, sugar, vegetable oils and trans fats. There is also some interesting evidence beginning to emerge that indicates that as 'third world' countries adopt the eating habits of the west instead of becoming healthier, their inflammatory markers increase and they actually become sicker and begin developing some of the chronic diseases of the Western World.

When we look at pro and anti inflammatory foods the most important thing to remember is that inflammation is an essential part of a healthy immune response. A healthy balanced diet should provide everything we need to support it, but if you suffer from gout or other inflammatory diseases your body is inflamed so you need to focus on a diet that is more anti than pro inflammatory. However, this does not mean that you have to stop eating food that promotes inflammation. Having a good balance of the right fats, proteins and carbohydrates is the key issue. Being liberal with your use of herbs and spices is a very simple way of boosting the anti-inflammatory potential of your food. To a certain extent herbs and spices are a 'secret weapon' when it comes to treating inflammation, especially as they are inexpensive and add an interesting and different dimension to our food. But, and this is a big but, they are not a wonder food. They may provide many of the trace elements, minerals and micronutrients our body's antioxidant defence teams needs, and they many have very powerful antioxidant and anti-inflammatory properties, but they can not make a bad diet good.

Allergies & Food Intolerance.

Common allergens are quick to spark an inflammatory cascade. Without wishing to sound cranky, one of the reasons you suffer from gout and have a body that is in a state of inflammation could be that you are unknowingly 'intolerant' of as opposed to allergic to some of the foods you consume on a regular basis. As a consequence these foods could be contributing to a state of systemic inflammation; wheat gluten, eggs, soy, dairy and some types of nuts, especially peanuts, are known allergens.

Lactose intolerance in particular is far more common than we realise. Figures vary but between 5% and 20% of people of Caucasian descent have a level of lactose intolerance. Around 35% of the South Sea Islanders have the problem. In people of African decent the figure rises to between 65% and 75%, while in some Asian populations the figures is as high as 90%.

Surprisingly tomatoes are also somewhat suspect. Some people can have an adverse reaction to tomatoes and other members of what is called "the nightshade" family of plants. Aubergines (egg plants), peppers and potatoes are also in this group. The adverse reaction is probably due to a substance called solanine that these vegetables contain. Some people believe that tomatoes can actually trigger an attack of gout.

Current research estimates that according to the International Foundation for Functional Gastrointestinal Disorders between 10% and 15% of the population suffer from symptoms of Irritable Bowel Syndrome, (IBS) that is triggered by a sensitivity to one or more specific foods. About 1% of the population of the developed world suffer from coeliac disease, an allergic auto immune condition that is associated with the consumption of grains like wheat and barley that contain gluten. True coeliac disease and gluten allergy at one end of the spectrum only affects a small minority of people but at the other end of the spectrum there are people who are sensitive to but not actually allergic to gluten. Notwithstanding this the sensitivity can create an inflammatory response. Unlike coeliac disease gluten sensitivity does not have any biomarkers so it can only be diagnosed by first ruling out other diseases and then trying a gluten free diet. Some researchers on gluten sensitivity estimate that around 6% of people of European decent have some degree of gluten sensitivity.

The bottom line is that with the typical Western diet we push our bodies too far. If you suspect that you are sensitive to a specific food or group of foods try eliminating it for at least two weeks. Listen to your body and see if symptoms like lethargy, headaches, 'foggy mind' depression, flatulence or bloating subside. Tedious and time consuming it may be but it is worth it in the long term. One last thing about food sensitivities is that as we get older foods that never bothered us before, like dairy and wheat, may trigger chronic low grade indigestion or other seemingly minor symptoms that can put our immune system onto high alert.

If you do decide to try an exclusion diet be mindful that they are not risk free. Many people with eating disorders begin with an exclusion diet that spirals out of control. The end result is anxiety and stress, both of which are entirely counter productive to treating gout and inflammation.

The Grain Debate

There is no doubt that as well as having the potential to cause allergies and food sensitivities, wheat and most other cereal grains are highly inflammatory foods. The more hybridised and processed the grain is the greater its inflammatory potential. Whole grains are the least inflammatory of the grains but in some people they can still cause inflammation and trigger an immune reaction.

The regular consumption of grain began about 10,000 years ago with the advent of the Agricultural Revolution. Before then man ate carbohydrate rich roots and tubers and gathered what grains and seeds he could when they were available. They ate them in very small amounts and they ate them whole and totally unrefined. Today edible grains make up the majority of the world's cultivated crops and they provide the greatest percentage of the calories consumed worldwide.

Grains and cereals are now in the middle of a sort of public relations nightmare with many people claiming major health benefits by adopting grain free diets. Some people actually go as far as to say that grains and cereals are toxic. Are grains good for us or are they bad? Well, all whole grains and cereals contain things that could potentially be bad for us but when grains are refined most of these are taken out during the milling process. One of the things that is often cited is Phytic Acid, something that can block the absorption of trace elements like calcium, iron and zinc, things that our bodies need. However, what the anti grain lobby fail to tell us is that there are many other foods that also contain phytic acid and consuming even modest amounts of sugary soft drinks can have the effect of actually 'leaching out' these same trace elements.

As well as gluten most grains and cereals also contain anti-nutrients like lectins and saponins, substances that can interfere with the absorption of nutrients. Some advocates of a grain free diet believe that these anti-nutrients act as toxins in our bodies. However, almost all food derived from plants contain anti-nutrients in one form or another as they are the plants' natural defences against pests, diseases and environmental threats. Tubers like potatoes are no exception. Most tubers are relatively toxic if eaten raw and a green potato, even when cooked, is actually quite poisonous.

Many believe that lectins and saponins can impair or damage the lining of the intestine and lead to digestive problems or food sensitivities. However, lectins are present in varying amounts in most foods. Most of the lectins we eat become harmless when they are cooked, but some can still be active when we eat them and interestingly, this type of lectin is usually found in grains and cereals. Notwithstanding this foods like carrots, apples and bananas also contain them and we eat most of these raw. As with so many things lectins become an issue when they are consumed in large amounts.

In the grain debate gluten is the key issue as it is known to be a major allergen that can cause severe inflammation in the small minority of people who are unable to digest it. But not all grains contain gluten; amaranth, buckwheat, corn, millet, most oats, quinoa and rice are all gluten free so should they be excluded from the grain debate?.

Interestingly some of the latest research into coeliac disease and gluten allergy suggests that something other than gluten could be the cause of coeliac disease. FODMAPS (Fermentable Oligo-Di-Monosaccharides and Polysols) are attracting a lot of attention and surprisingly quite a large number of people are sensitive to them. FODMAPS are present in a large number of foods in varying amounts, legumes, cows milk, soft cheese, yoghurt, fruit and vegetables, including apples, mangos, onions and garlic just to name a few contain them. However, FODMAPS are low in oats, spelt and soy sauce and interestingly these are things that are not usually allowed in a gluten free diet. To certain extent the jury is out on gluten as evidence is beginning to emerge that FODMAPS could be causing the problem. Gluten could be an innocent bystander

The consumption of grains and cereals is fast becoming a big issue. Part of the controversy about gluten free and gluten sensitivity is that we are being sold a lot of misinformation. Several best selling books have been highly influential in steering healthy people away from the 'dangers' of wheat and gluten by making generalisations and exaggerated claims. Some go as far as to say that gluten and carbohydrates are destroying our brains!

Some prominent people have treated genuine physiological conditions themselves by excluding gluten from their diet and the media coverage has meant that their stories have snowballed. Now more and more people are taking the view that '*if it works for them it must be worth giving it a go*'. Enter the placebo effect and for many it becomes difficult to disentangle the benefits they may experience by adopting a gluten free diet from their expectation that the change in their diet will make them feel better.

The grain debate is having a major impact on public opinion which, according to Mintel, is split between 41% of people in the United States who think that gluten free diets are of benefit and 44% who think they are a fad. A recent survey found that 29% of adult Americans, 70 million people, were trying to cut back on their consumption of gluten. In the UK the polster YouGov reported that 60% of adults have at some time purchased a gluten free product and that 10% of households, over 2½ million homes, include someone who believes that gluten is bad for them.

Enter the food manufacturing industry which has quickly cottoned on to 'gluten free' as being the latest marketing ploy with projected revenue in the United States estimated to increase from $8.8bn in 2014 to $14.2bn in 2017. In the UK new product launches of 'healthy' gluten free snack bars has increased from 25% in 2013 to 40% in 2014.

Why have our views on the consumption of grains changed so rapidly? Some people have suggested that the increased interest in a gluten free diet has little to do with public awareness of coeliac disease and gluten sensitivity but a lot to do with the popularity of diets that are aimed at moving us back to the type of hunter gatherer food our early ancestors are thought to have consumed. Others see it as connecting these myths about man's early diet with an increasing "anti" attitude to the food manufacturing industry. One thing is certain however, with the food manufacturing industry now focused on a new rapidly growing sector, with increased advertising and promotional activity "gluten free" and the grain debate is destined to become quite a hot topic.

Are we simply eating too many grains?

The ability to grow and process grains and cereals more easily allowed people to eat more of them. The bottom line is that we are simply eating too many grains and cereals and the ones we are eating are in the wrong form; refined grains for breakfast in our cereal, refined grains for lunch in some form of bread, may be a muffin at some time of the day as a snack and probably more refined grains in the evening as pasta or pizza.

From an evolutionary perspective the 10,000 years since the Agricultural Revolution is no where near long enough for our digestive capacity to evolve sufficiently enough to be able to consume the high concentrations of refined grains and cereals that is found in our diet today. But this change in diet has not happened over thousands of years. Up until fairly recent history only the rich could afford to eat flour that was in any way refined and 'white'. As you went down through the social scale less wheat and more rye and oatmeal was consumed and the coarser and less refined this 'flour' became. By the time you got to the really poor, they could not afford flour at all. They ate a sort of meal made from ground up beans and pulses, the equivalent of current day gram (chickpea) flour.

Historically carbohydrates generally were in short supply. There were no potatoes and there was no rice. The carbohydrates that were available were all complex and unrefined. Sugar was an extremely expensive luxury, as was honey, and only the rich could afford to buy it. With the exception of small amounts of fruit that could be dried or stored, fruit was seasonal. Only the rich could afford the sugar or honey needed to preserve it.

The jury is still out on the grain debate. It depends to a certain extent on which side of the fence you are sitting. Consuming grains may be right for some people and wrong for others. If you do eat them focus on quality and processing techniques, eat smaller amounts and only eat 'whole' grains. Eat more vegetables and non grain sources of carbohydrates whenever you can. Eating a balanced diet and cutting back on something that is known to be inflammatory can only be a good thing.

To Fry Or Not To Fry?

If you are eating to treat gout and inflammation the simple answer is do not fry your food. At the very least limit your consumption of fried food to just once in a while.

One of the intriguing aspects of the 'Western Diet' is the high heat at which so much of our food is cooked. We fry food in fat or oil, we grill it, we BBQ it and we roast and bake it in hot ovens. We seem to be addicted to browned, caramelised and crisp food. The effect that these cooking methods have on our food is immense and the nutritional content and chemical structure of our food both suffer. Cooking at high temperatures can transform otherwise healthy foods into unhealthy compounds that can cause serious damage to our bodies and as a consequence our heath. What these compounds are and precisely how they damage our health is not the subject of this book but the oil we use to cook the food in is.

When any oil or fat is heated to high temperatures the oil oxidises and free radicals are produced, often in large numbers. Some of these are very aggressive free radicals that can set off chain reactions that have the potential to damage some of the cells in our bodies. The need to neutralise these free radicals puts an increased load on our body's anti-oxidant defences. Chemicals called aldehydes and lipid peroxides are also produced when oil and fat is heated. These are extremely damaging substances and consuming or inhaling them even in small amounts has been linked to cancer and heart disease. Both of them can damage and kill cells and when this happens the resulting trauma increases inflammation as well as the amount of uric acid in your body.

Cooking at high temperatures and frying in particular is basically not a good idea as all fried food is highly inflammatory but if we accept the fact that we are going to fry food which oils and fats should we be using?

All oils and fats oxidise when they are heated and exposed to sunlight. The more polyunsaturated the fat or oil is the more it oxidises. The more saturated the fat is the less it oxidises. For years we have been told that frying with vegetable oils is healthier than cooking with animal fat like butter or lard, but is it? Oils like sunflower and corn oil that are rich in polyunsaturates generate the highest levels of aldehydes and lipid peroxides when they are used for frying and cooking. In contrast olive oil and cold pressed rapeseed oil produce far less aldehydes as do butter, lard and goose fat. The reason for this is that these oils are richer in saturated and monounsaturated fatty acids than the polyunsaturated oils and the monounsaturated and saturated fatty acids are much more stable when they are heated. In fact saturated fats generate hardly any aldehydes or lipid peroxides when they are heated.

Corn oil and sunflower oil are loaded with polyunsaturated fats; corn oils contains 54% and sunflower oil 65%. While it contains 63% monounsaturated fats rape seed oil also contains 28% polyunsaturated fats and these are not in a particularly good Omega-3 to Omega-6 ratio. So the general recommendation is to use olive oil for frying or cooking as it contains about 76% monounsaturated, 14% saturated and only 10% polyunsaturated fats. As the monounsaturated and saturated fats are much more resistant to oxidation than the polyunsaturated fats this means that they produce lower levels of aldehydes and lipid peroxides as well as fewer free radicals. In addition the compounds that are generated are far less damaging to the body. When it comes to cooking with olive oil it makes no difference whether you use hot or cold pressed oil as there are not enough anti-oxidants in the cold pressed oil to protect it from heat induced oxidation.

After years of being told that saturated fat is bad for us quite a lot of evidence is beginning to emerge that eating some saturated fats may actually help you loose weight and also be good for your heart. So another option is to use butter, lard and goose fat for cooking as they are all much better than polyunsaturated oils.

If you are eating to treat gout and inflammation the best advice is to eat less fried food, especially food that has been cooked at high temperatures. All fried food, irrespective of what type of oil it is fried in, is also very high in calories. If you do fry food minimise the amount of oil or fat that you use and drain the food well on kitchen paper before you eat it. It is also advisable to store your oils is the dark as sunlight accelerates the speed at which they oxidise. Do not reuse fats and oils. This leads to the accumulation of free radicals, aldehydes and lipid peroxides and this makes them even more unhealthy fats and oils.

Gout, Inflammation & Our Diet

Like many things in life food can be addictive and manufactured and processed foods really are addictive, the food manufacturers have made sure of that. Dietary habits are just that, habits, and like all habits they can be changed. However, urging someone to change the eating habits of a lifetime is no easy task. It is a fact that less than 20% of patients seeking medical advice are able or prepared to make substantial lifestyle and dietary changes. In the management and treatment of gout and inflammation, making dietary and lifestyle changes are the two most important things you can do to help yourself.

If you suffer from gout your body is inflamed and it is not functioning properly. In order to get it back into proper working order, the essential first step towards leading a gout and inflammation free life, you need a long term solution. There is no magic cure and there are no silver bullets. For years the gout and inflammation disease sufferer has been told that cherry juice, apple cider vinegar, bicarbonate of soda, red cabbage, tablets of green tea and special food supplements were the wonder foods that would cure their diseases. The sad reality is that you cannot rectify a diet that is overloaded with the wrong foods and completely lacking in the essential vitamins, minerals, antioxidants and Omega-3 fats it so desperately needs by simply taking a one off cure. We need to look at the 'big picture' and correct the underlying causes of gout and inflammation.

The truth about what causes gout and a diet that is designed to treat gout and inflammation is explained in full in Goodbye To Gout. - A New Gout Diet. This is not a diet in the typical meaning of the word as there are no meal plans and there is no calorie counting. It is more of an eating, cooking and food selection programme that is designed to help you eat wisely. It is a set of guidelines as opposed to a set of strict rules. It is all about making a switch from the foods that can cause gout and inflammation to the foods that will restore your body's natural balance and set you on the road to recovery. The occasional mishap won't spell doom. It is what you do 'most of the time', not what you do 'some of the time' that matters and, unlike some rigidly restrictive diets, it does not take the fun out of eating. You don't have to give up eggs and butter or any of the other foods high in purines that have for so long been unjustly given a bad press.

This diet is essentially an 'Always, Sometimes and Never' eat diet; there is some food that you can always eat because it helps to reduce inflammation and it does not cause gout, some food you can sometimes eat or eat in moderation because it is only slightly inflammatory and some food that you should never eat, simply because it can cause gout and it fuels inflammation.

What are the foods you can always, sometimes and never eat?

The food you can ALWAYS eat:

- Vegetables, Pulses and Fruit
- Fish, especially oily cold water fish, and seafood
- Herbs, Spices, Nuts and Seeds
- Dairy Products, especially low fat dairy products
- Eggs
- Tofu, Soya Bean Curd and Tempeh
- Olive Oil
- Dark Chocolate and Cocoa
- White, Green , Oolong Tea and plenty of Water
- Butter and other Saturated Fats

The food you can SOMETIMES eat:

- Whole Grain Carbohydrates; Oatmeal, Quinoa, Millet, Buckwheat, Bulgar Wheat, Spelt and Barley
- The Humble Potato
- Pasta
- Rice and Rice Noodles
- Coffee and Red Wine

The food you should NEVER eat:

- Polyunsaturated Vegetable Oils and Trans Fats
- Refined Carbohydrates
- Sugar and High Fructose Corn Syrup
- Alcohol; Beer, Lager, Cider, White Wine and Spirits
- Food that contains iron
- Food that is fried, grilled and roasted at high temperatures
- Fruit juice and smoothies.

This probably looks like quite a challenge. Put simply eating to treat gout and inflammation is about going back to basics, and unless you can find a safe and reliable source of healthy manufactured foods this means cooking.

Can't cook, haven't got time to cook, don't know how to cook? It is not as hard as you think. After all it is only over the last fifty to sixty years that we have stopped cooking. Taking back control of cooking could well be the single most important step you take on the road to recovery. Reclaiming cooking will provide you with healthier food, it will make you self reliant and it will open a door to a more enjoyable and nourishing life. But before we start cooking, we need to look at the kitchen and the store cupboard.

The Kitchen & The Store Cupboard

Cooking at home requires some advance planning and preparation. If you do not already 'cook' here are some tips on how to begin.

Kitchen Equipment

A well equipped kitchen saves time and effort and it can take much of the drudgery out of the preparation of food. Kitchen tools and equipment come in a many different options, ranging from basic and manual to fully automatic with all the bells and whistles.

You know the basics; sharp knives, cutting boards, spatulas, pots and pans, measuring cups and spoons etc. but there are other tools and appliances that are 'nice to have' rather than essential. Here are a few of our favourite 'essential' kitchen tools that will make life in the kitchen that much easier.

A Handheld (stick) Blender

With chopping/blending and whisk attachments. You can use this to blend soup, purée and whiz ingredients together and whisk egg whites.

A Food Processor
For slicing, grating, chopping and general mixing. You may be able to manage quite well with only a very small one but you will find a machine with a 2½ Litre/4¼ pint/10 cup bowl the most useful.

Blender
If you feel unable to stretch to a food processor a small blender will help with some of the chopping and blending tasks.

Coffee Grinder:
Reserved for grinding spices as spices taste much better when they are freshly ground.

Pestle and Mortar
As an alternative for grinding spices and making pestos,

Silicon Bakeware
I am a great convert to silicon bakeware so if you have not already invested in conventional baking tins buy some silicon baking equipment As a suggestion it is worth investing in

- a 1.4Lt/2½ pt loaf tin,
- a 20cm/8 in square cake tin,
- a 24cm/10 in diameter round cake tin,
- some 150ml/5 fl oz (¼ pt) muffin tins and
- a silicon baking mat.

A Potato Ricer
Not strictly essential but useful as it 'mashes' things without turning them into a mush.

Cooking Pans
You will find a non stick 24cm/10in frying pan or chef's pan (with a lid) that can go in the oven as well as on the hob, a wok and some non stick saucepans very useful.

The Store Cupboard

For most of us, whether it is because of convenience or simple economics, shopping in supermarkets is an inevitable part of our life. As well as fruit and vegetables they are a good place to stock up on canned and frozen food and the things you need to buy in large quantities. Farmers markets, speciality markets, ethnic markets and on line retailers often carry the harder to find ingredients that your local supermarkets does no stock. Whatever you buy and wherever you buy it remember to read the labels so that you know exactly what is in the food you are buying. If you can find the time, grow some things yourself, especially herbs and sprouting seeds like mustard cress and alfalfa. You don't need a lot of land - pots take up very little space and nothing tastes better than something you have grown yourself.

In addition to fresh ingredients you need a well stocked pantry. Don't forget the freezer. Here is a list of some of the ingredients you will need to have on hand as you cook your way through the recipes in this book.

Herbs:

Most fresh herbs will keep in the fridge for up to a week if they are wrapped in kitchen paper and stored in a box. They also keep well in a jar of water on the window sill. Better still, buy growing herbs. Basil, parsley and coriander do well in pots and a small bay plant on the window sill is very useful. Herbs also freeze well - see the recipes for making different types of pesto, and freezing herbs does not affect their nutritional value. Making your own pesto and keeping a supply in the freezer is well worth the effort. Drying herbs is another option but with the exception of dill and rosemary, most dried herbs just don't taste the same as fresh ones.

Because they have powerful anti-inflammatory properties the recipes in this book use a lot of ginger and chilli. You can buy frozen grated ginger and frozen chopped chilli. As with different types of pesto you will find a stock of this in the freezer very useful.

Spices:

It is best to buy whole spices as once they are ground they begin to loose their flavour quickly. A coffee grinder reserved for spices works well or you can use a simple pestle and mortar. Whether they are whole or ground, store spices away from heat, light and moisture and replace them every six months. A list of some of the less common spices that you need to look out for:-

Tamarind: used extensively in Asian cooking. It gives food a characteristic tart, sour flavour.

Sumac: a Middle Eastern spice with a sharp slightly sour taste.

Chilli: as well as whole fresh chillies you can use chilli as a paste, ground into a fine powder or very finely chopped as in Sambol Oelek.

Turmeric: This has very strong anti-inflammatory properties.. If you are lucky enough to be able to buy this fresh do so, otherwise you will need to rely on dried powdered turmeric.

Garam Masala: A useful Asian blend of spices.

Garlic: Another strongly anti-inflammatory ingredient. As well as fresh garlic, stock up on dried garlic granules and if you an find them some smoked dried garlic granules.

Healthy fats and oils:

Make sure you have a supply of healthy fats and oils; cold pressed olive oil, butter and, if you can buy it, clarified butter or Ghee. Store the olive oil in the dark or in the fridge to slow down the rate at which it oxidises.

Miscellaneous Ingredients

- Wholegrain Spelt. An 'old' type of grain that is the same family as wheat. It contains less gluten than wheat and is a healthy alternative to conventional whole grain flour.
- Flaked and fine oatmeal. You can usually find flaked or rolled oats in your local supermarket but fine oatmeal, sometimes referred to as pin head oatmeal, is more difficult to obtain. You can make your

own by processing a batch of flaked oats in a blender or food processor until the oats look like a coarse flour. Store the fine oatmeal in an airtight jar.

- Dried Porchini mushrooms or dried Ceps.
- Truffle oil, an expensive luxury that is well worth the investment.
- Preserved lemons; used in Middle Eastern and North African cooking. Use lemon rind soaked for half and hour in brine if you are unable to get them.
- Miso paste: either as white miso or brown miso and used extensively in Japanese cooking, If has a strong fermented taste.
- Thai Fish Sauce. It contains a lot of salt but if you are not otherwise adding salt to your cooking, once in a while it's OK.
- Sesame Oil.
- Vegetable stock cubes or vegetable stock powder.
- Tahini, a paste made from ground sesame seeds.
- Japanese Panko Breadcrumbs; yes they are made from wheat but they are very useful when used in small amounts.

Reading Recipes

If you are new to cooking start by reading all the way through a recipe before you begin making it. Don't be put off by a long list of ingredients. A long list of ingredients does not necessarily mean that a recipe is going to be difficult.

Make sure you give yourself enough time to cook without feeling pressured or rushed. Being stressed about cooking is counter productive. As you gain experience and confidence in the kitchen you will be amazed at how quickly you can get a meal cooked and on the table. Be prepared for some things not to turn out as you expected and for some recipes not to be to your liking. The more you cook the more comfortable you will become and the more confident you will be with changing recipes to suit your personal taste. Remember, a recipe is a guide not a rigid process.

PART FOUR

THE RECIPE COLLECTION

Home cooked food nourishes the soul as well as the body but we need to be realistic about it. Time and energy are precious, especially during the working week. Here is a selection of recipes that can be prepared in advance or made when you have limited time to cook, Many of them can also be frozen or made with ingredients from the freezer. The recipes taste good, they can be eaten by the whole family and they all have a place in an anti-inflammatory diet

A cookbook without pictures! You can go to

goodbye-to-gout.com/recipe_pics

to see what the recipes look like. Not all the recipes are in the photo gallery but it is growing all the time.

CONTENTS

SOUPS & CHOWDERS

Why so many recipes for soup? If you suffer from gout you need to keep yourself hydrated, so because soups contain a lot of water they play an important part in a gout diet.

Soups are less complicated to make than many people imagine. Some of the best classic soups are simply vegetables that are cooked gently in olive oil or butter, then simmered until tender and sieved, mashed or liquidised. Cream, milk or yoghurt and fresh herbs add a special touch. With a few exceptions soups can usually be frozen, so it is worthwhile making twice the quantity and building up a supply of your own 'fast food'.

It is easy to make your own vegetable stock and it freezes well but if you do not have time to do this you can use any good quality vegetable stock or vegetable stock powder.

CONTENTS

English Onion Soup

This soup scores high on the anti inflammation scale and it is also a really simple soup to make. The dry vermouth and grated raw onion added at the end give it an extra special twist. If you have some truffle oil just a small amount sprinkled on when the soup is served tastes amazing.

The soup freezes well and can be stored in the fridge for up to 2 days.

SERVES 4

700g/1 lb 9 oz onions peeled and thinly sliced

2 tbsp grated onion

400g/14oz potatoes peeled and sliced

3 tbsp olive oil

1.7Lt/3pt vegetable stock

4 tbsp dry vermouth (optional)

4 tbsp fromage frais or natural unsweetened yoghurt

¼ tsp grated nutmeg

salt and pepper to taste

4 tbsp grated parmesan to serve OR some truffle oil

1   Heat the olive oil in a large saucepan and add the sliced onions and the potato. Sauté them for 5 minutes and then add the stock. Bring to the boil, cover, reduce the heat and simmer them for 20 minutes until the potatoes and onions are tender.

2   Use a hand blender to blend the soup until it is smooth. Add the dry vermouth if you are using it and season to taste with the grated nutmeg, salt and black pepper.

3   When you are ready to serve the soup stir in the grated onion and fromage frais. Serve the grated Parmesan in a separate bowl.

Thai Carrot Soup

Yellow Thai curry is made from chillies, turmeric, ginger and garlic. As all of these are strongly anti-inflammatory, a yellow Thai curry or curry soup makes a healthy anti-inflammatory meal. You can buy Thai curry paste on line and in Asian supermarkets. If you want to make your own, a recipe is included in the Herbs and Spices section.

This soup freezes well and can be kept in the fridge for up to 2 days.

SERVES 4

1 large white onion finely sliced
1 tbsp olive oil
700g/1 lb 8 oz carrots
1Lt/35 fl oz vegetable stock

100g/3½oz red lentils
1 tbsp yellow Thai curry paste
3 handfuls of coriander finely chopped

1 Peel and slice the carrots into 5ml/¼in rounds.

2 Heat the olive oil over a medium heat and add the onion. Sauté for a minute or two. Add the Thai curry paste and the sliced carrots and stir for a minute or two.

3 Add the vegetable stock and the lentils. Turn up the heat and bring the soup to the boil, stirring occasionally to prevent the lentils sticking.

4 Turn the heat to low, cover and simmer for 30 minutes.

5 When you are ready to serve, blitz the soup with a hand blender and stir in half of the chopped coriander. Serve the rest of the coriander in a separate bowl.

Roasted Pumpkin Soup

You can use pumpkin or butternut squash to make this. Serve the soup
with lightly toasted pumpkin seeds.

SERVES 4 – 6

1Kg/2 lb 4oz pumpkin, peeled and cut into chunks

8 cloves of garlic unpeeled

2 tbsp olive oil

White of 3 leeks finely sliced

1Lt/1¾ pt/35 fl oz vegetable stock

½ tsp grated nutmeg

1 large eating apple peeled and cut into chunks

4 tbsp fromage frais or natural unsweetened yoghurt

2 tbsp finely chopped parsley

2 tbsp lightly toasted pumpkin seeds

Pre heat the oven to 200°C/ 400°F/Gas 5.

1   Put the pumpkin and garlic onto a baking tray lined with non stick foil. Drizzle over 1 tablespoon of the olive oil and roast for 30 minutes.

2   Heat the remaining tablespoon of olive oil in a large saucepan. Add the sliced leeks and the apple and sauté for 5 minutes. Add the stock and grated nutmeg, bring to the boil and simmer over a low heat while the pumpkin cooks.

3   When the pumpkin and garlic is cooked squeeze the garlic into the stock and leeks and then add the roasted pumpkin. Bring the soup back to the boil, turn off the heat and blend it with a hand blender until it is smooth and creamy.

4   Just before serving stir in the fromage frais or yoghurt and sprinkle on the chopped parsley.

Borscht

There are many recipes for this classic beetroot soup. Some are thickened and served hot, some are thin and clear, almost like a consomée, and served cold. You can serve this as a soup or with various different accompaniments as part of a main meal.

SERVES 6

1kg/2¼ lb fresh or cooked beetroot

1.3Lt/2¼pt vegetable stock

2 tbsp olive oil

1 large onion, about 200g/7oz, peeled an sliced

450g/1 lb potatoes peeled and cut into 1cm/½ in slices

100g/3½oz carrots peeled and cut

3 cloves crushed garlic

Zest and juice of a lemon

To Serve

150ml/5 fl oz natural Greek yoghurt

3 - 4 tbsp finely chopped spring onions

2 tbsp chopped dill

2 hard boiled eggs finely chopped

1   If the beetroot are raw cover them with water, bring them to the boil and simmer for 1 hour. Drain them, refresh them on cold water and peel them. Cut the beetroot into 2cm/1 inch chunks.

2   Sauté the onions in the oil for a couple of minutes and then add the potatoes and carrots. Stir them around for one or two minutes and then add the beetroot, the crushed garlic and the lemon zest. Pour on the vegetable stock, bring to the boil, cover and simmer for 20 minutes.

3   Turn off the heat and blitz the soup using a hand blender. Just before serving stir in the lemon juice. Serve with the yogurt, chopped dill, herbs, spring onions and chopped hard boiled eggs in separate bowls.

Gazpacho

This summer soup needs no cooking. You can prepare it in advance and keep it for up to 24 hours in the fridge.

SERVES 4

1 medium red onion	2tbsp red wine vinegar
1 red or green pepper de-seeded	2tbsp olive oil
½ large telegraph cucumber	salt and freshly ground black pepper
500g/1 lb ripe vine tomatoes	1 large tomato to garnish
60g/2oz stale white bread	To Serve
2 cloves of garlic crushed	Tabasco, Tahini and basil pesto

1   First you need to peel the tomatoes. Put them in a bowl and cover them with boiling water. Leave them for about a minute and then plunge them into ice cold water. The skins will have split and they will peel off quite easily.

2   Cut the onion, pepper and cucumber into large chunks. Put them into a food processor or blender and process them for a few seconds. Try to keep the texture fairly chunky. Transfer a quarter of the chopped vegetables to a bowl, cover the bowl and refrigerate. These vegetables will be used later as a garnish.

3   Add the tomatoes, bread, garlic vinegar and olive oil to the remainder of the vegetables in the food processor and blend once more. If the soup looks a little thick add some cold water. Season with salt and pepper, cover and place in the fridge to chill.

4   When you are ready to serve the soup finely chop the remaining tomato and add it to the bowl of reserved vegetables. Ladle the soup into a large serving bowl. Serve the vegetables in a separate bowl with some Tabasco, Tahini and basil pesto.

Mussel, Leek & Saffron Soup

This recipe uses frozen mussels as they take less time to prepare and are widely available in supermarkets. You can also use fresh mussels in their shells if you can get them. If you do use fresh mussels you will need about 1.5Kg/3lb.

SERVES 4

300g/11oz frozen mussel meat, thawed, washed and dried

450g/16oz leeks coarsely chopped

5cm/2in piece white part of a leek cut into match stick size pieces

50ml/2 fl oz white wine OR Noilly Prat (optional)

1 small onion chopped

50g/2oz butter

1tbsp flour

450ml/15 fl oz fish stock OR

450ml/15fl oz vegetable stock and 1Tbsp Thai fish sauce

A large pinch of saffron

50ml/2 fl oz fromage frais or natural unsweetened Greek yoghurt

1   Melt the butter in a saucepan and sauté the leeks and onion on a medium heat for 3 - 4 minutes. Be careful not to let them brown.

2   Stir in the flour and cook for 2 minutes. Add the stock and the saffron. If using vegetable stock and Thai fish sauce add the fish sauce just before you serve the soup. Bring everything to the boil, turn down the heat and simmer for 25 - 30 minutes.

3   Use a hand blender to purée the leeks and onion. At this stage you can turn off the heat or leave the soup simmering on a low heat.

4   When you are ready to serve the soup add the mussels, bring the soup to the boil and simmer gently for 5 minutes. Don't overcook the mussels as they will become tough.

5   Just before serving stir in the cream or yoghurt. Ladle the soup into individual bowls and garnish with the slices of leek.

Ginger, Noodle & Mushroom Soup

This recipe uses soba noodles that are made from buckwheat but you can use any type of egg or rice noodles. If you use dried shitake mushrooms follow the rehydration and cooking instructions on the packet.

SERVES 4

200g/7oz chestnut mushrooms cut into 5mm/¼ in slices OR 15g/½oz dried shitake mushrooms

1Lt/1¾ pt/35 fl oz vegetable stock

125g/4½ oz soba noodles

2 tbsp olive oil

3 cloves of garlic finely chopped

1 tsp Sambol Oelek or ½ tsp chilli powder

2 tbsp grated ginger

1 tsp light soy sauce

125g/4½oz bean sprouts washed and drained OR finely sliced Chinese leaf

Roughly chopped coriander to garnish

1   Bring a saucepan of water to the boil. Add the soba noodles and cook following the instructions on the packet. This is usually about 8 minutes. Drain and stir in a small amount of olive oil to stop the noodles sticking together. Put them to one side while you cook the mushrooms.

2   Heat the oil in a saucepan and sauté the mushrooms over a medium heat for 2 to 3 minutes. Add the garlic and ginger and cook for another 2 minutes.

3   Add the vegetable stock, the chilli and soy sauce and bring to the boil. Add the bean sprouts and bring the stock back to the boil, then add the cooked noodles and heat them through.

4   Serve garnished with the coriander.

Curried Parsnip Soup

This is a thick chunky soup that is somewhere between a Chowder and a soup. Serve it on its own or with a cucumber raita.

Like all soups this can be frozen and kept for up to 3 months. You can freeze it with or without the cooked barley.

SERVES 4

100g/3½oz pearly barley
700g/1½lbs parsnips, peeled
1 large white onion finely chopped
1 large desert apple cored a roughly chopped
1 stick of celery finely chopped
1 tbsp olive oil
1½ Lt/2¼ pt vegetable stock
1 tsp garlic powder
2½cm/1 in piece ginger grated
1 red chilli finely chopped OR 1 tsp Sambol Oelek

2 tsp ground coriander
1 tsp ground cumin
½ tsp ground fenugreek
½ tsp turmeric

For the cucumber raita
250g/9oz natural unsweetened yoghurt
½ telegraph cucumber
1 clove garlic crushed
1 tsp dried dill

1   Wash the pearl barley in several changes of water. Put it into a saucepan, cover it with plenty of water and bring it to the boil. Do not add any salt as this tends to prevent the barley from cooking properly. Cover, turn the heat down to very low and leave the barley to simmer for 50 - 60 minutes. By this time the barley should be tender.

2   Strain the barley and rinse it in cold water. You can do this in advance of making the soup. You can keep the cooked barley in the fridge in a covered container for 2 or 3 days. It also freezes well for up to 3 months.

3   Remove the core from the parsnips and chop them into even size

chunks. If the parsnips are small you can leave the cores in.

4   Heat the olive oil in a large saucepan, add the finely chopped onion and sauté lightly over a medium heat for a minute or two.

5   Add the chopped parsnips, the celery and the apple. Give everything a good stir, then add the spices and grated ginger. Cook for 2 minutes stirring all the time and then add the vegetable stock, Bring everything to the boil, cover, turn down the heat to low and simmer for 30 minutes.

6   To make the cucumber raita. Place a tea towel or a piece of muslin on a deep plate and coarsely grate the cucumber onto it. Gather up the material and squeeze out as much of the fluid from the cucumber as you can. You will be amazed how much comes out. Stir this fluid into the soup.

7   Put the cucumber into a bowl and add ½ a clove of crushed garlic and the dried dill. Give it a good stir and then add about two thirds of the yoghurt. Stir it round and if the mixture looks too thick add the rest of the yoghurt. How much you need to add depends on how much fluid was left in the cucumber.

8   When the soup has finished cooking take it off the heat and blend it with a hand blender. Stir in the cooked pearly barley and heat through. Serve the soup in individual bowls with a spoonful of the cucumber raita swirled into the top.

Tomato & Lentil Soup

This is a basic soup that you can easily transform into something completely different by simply changing the herbs and spices you use.

SERVES 4

400g/14oz tin chopped tomatoes

3 tbsp tomato purée

1 large red onion roughly chopped

1 stick celery roughly chopped

1 large carrot roughly chopped

100g/3½oz red lentils

1 tbsp olive oil

1tsp Sambol Oelek or ½ tsp chilli powder (optional)

700ml/25 fl oz/1¼pt vegetable stock

3 cloves of garlic roughly chopped

4 tbsp natural unsweetened Greek style yoghurt

handful of torn basil leaves

1 Wash and pick over the red lentils and make sure that there is no grit in them. Leave them to drain while you prepare the vegetables.

2 Heat the olive oil and lightly sauté the onion, garlic, celery and carrot for 3 or 4 minutes. Don't let them brown. Add the tin of chopped tomatoes, the tomato purée, the Sambol Oelek and chilli.

3 Add the vegetable stock and the lentils. Give everything a good stir, bring it to the boil, cover and simmer for 30 - 40 minutes until the lentils are tender.

4 Using a hand blender blend the soup until it is smooth. Stir in the yoghurt and the torn basil leaves.

Variation: You can give this soup a Middle Eastern flavour by omitting the yoghurt and basil and adding 1 tsp ground cumin, 1 tsp dried dill and ½ tsp ground cardamom seeds when you add the tin of tomatoes.

Sweetcorn & Basil Soup

With sweetcorn, butter and cream as the main ingredients this is definitely a soup that comes into the 'sometimes eat' category. Why is it here? Simply because the combination of fresh basil, cream and sweetcorn is delicious.

You can use fresh or frozen sweetcorn to make this soup. It is best made with fresh corn that is on the cob but you can make a quicker version if you use frozen sweetcorn kernels. The soup can be served hot or cold. As with just about all soups it can be frozen but if you decide to freeze it leave out the basil and add it when you are going to eat the soup.

SERVES 4

4 large corn on the cob.	60ml/2 fl oz cream or fromage frais
50g/1½oz butter	A large bunch of basil
200g/7oz chopped white onion	
1.5Lt/2¼pt vegetable stock	

1 If the sweetcorn is frozen thaw it out by popping it into hot water for a few minutes.

2 Take the kernels of sweetcorn off of the cobs. Melt the butter, yes its a lot of butter but it really does add to the flavour. Add the chopped onion, lightly sauté it for a few minutes and then add the stock. Bring it to the boil and add the inside cobs of the sweetcorn. bring it back to the boil, cover and simmer for 30 minutes.

3 Take out the cobs and add the sweetcorn kernels. Bring the soup back to the boil, cover and simmer for 20 - 25 minutes until the sweetcorn is tender.

4 Turn off the heat and process the soup with a hand blender until it is smooth.

5 Now you need to pass the soup through a sieve. You don't have to

do this but sieving it gives the soup a much smoother and finer texture. Use a wooden spoon to push the mush of sweetcorn through the sieve. You will get a sort of thick purée on the underside of the sieve and you need to scrape this into the soup. Carry on doing this until the top of the sieve only contains coarse corn husks.

6   Stir in the cream and add the bunch of basil. Leave the basil to infuse for between 1 to 12 hours. When you are ready to serve the soup, take out the bunch of basil, scrape off any soup that is dripping from it and serve the soup either hot or cold.

7   The quick version: sauté the onion in the butter, add 1Lt/35 fl oz stock and then add 375g/12oz frozen sweetcorn. Cook as above and then purée the soup until it is as smooth as you can possibly get it, then stir in the cream and the bunch of basil. Leave the basil to infuse for at least an hour before serving.

Hot & Sour Soup With Watercress

A very easy soup that you can have ready in minutes. You can use any type of mushroom including dried mushrooms. Tamarind has a unique tart slightly sour flavour and is widely used in Asian cooking. You will find tamarind in Asian food stores and you can also buy it on line. Instructions on how to make the tamarind pulp are included in the section on Herbs and Spices. If you do not have any tamarind use lemon or lime juice instead.

SERVES 4

250g/9oz firm tofu dried and cut into 2cm/¾ in cubes
2 tbsp olive oil
100g/3½oz chestnut or shitake mushrooms sliced
2 tbsp chopped coriander
100g/3½oz watercress, large stems removed
1 red chilli finely sliced

For the stock:
2 tbsp tamarind pulp
2 dried red chillies
2 kafir lime leaves OR 2 tsp grated lime zest
2 tbsp grated ginger
1 onion cut into quarters
1Lt/1¾ pt/35 fl oz water

1 Put all of the ingredients for the stock into a saucepan,and bring them to the boil. Reduce the heat and simmer for 10 minutes.

2 While the stock is cooking heat 1 tbsp oil oil in a frying pan and sauté the mushrooms over a medium heat for 5 minutes. Remove and put to one side.

3 Add the rest of the oil to the frying pan and fry the tofu over a medium heat for 5 minutes turning it over to seal it on all sides.

4 Strain the stock and return it to the saucepan. Add the mushrooms and the watercress and bring the soup back to the boil. Stir in the sliced chilli and tofu and turn off the heat. Serve garnished with the chopped coriander.

Potato, Chestnut & Porcini Chowder

As with the curried parsnip soup this is more of a chowder than a soup. To make this you need firm, waxy new potatoes that will not disintegrate when they are cooked. The Porcini mushrooms are an essential ingredient. You can use frozen, tinned or vacuum packed chestnuts. The soup will not freeze.

SERVES 4

3 banana shallots finely chopped

20g/¾oz Porcini mushrooms

3 tbsp olive oil

1 tsp garlic powder

½ tsp cayenne pepper

½ tsp ground turmeric

2 tsp dried rosemary finely chopped

1Kg/2 lb 4oz small waxy new potatoes cut into 5mm/¼ in slices

1.5Lt/2¼pt vegetable stock

20 peeled and cooked chestnuts cut into quarters

90g/3oz finely grated parmesan

Crushed black pepper

Finely chopped parsley or chervil to garnish

1 Bring the vegetable stock to the boil and add the Porcini mushrooms, the cayenne pepper, garlic powder, turmeric and rosemary. Turn off the heat and leave them to soak for at least half an hour. Bring them to the boil and leave them simmering while you prepare the rest of the ingredients.

2 Heat the oil in a large saucepan and sauté the shallots for 2 or 3 minutes. Add the potatoes and sauté for a couple of minutes.

3 Add the chestnuts and the vegetable stock with the Porcini mushrooms. Bring to the boil, reduce the heat and simmer for 12 - 15 minutes until the potatoes are just tender. Turn off the heat and just before serving stir in the parmesan and black pepper. Garnish with finely chopped parsley or chervil.

Fennel & Salmon Chowder
This is a simple soup that is quick and easy to prepare.

SERVES 4

1 medium onion finely sliced

3 large or 4 small bulbs of fennel

2 tbsp olive oil

1 large potato peeled and cut into
1cm/½ in chunks

300g/10½oz salmon cut into
1cm/½ in pieces

Finely grated zest of ½ lemon

600ml/1 pt fish stock OR vegetable stock
plus 1 tbsp Thai fish sauce

Juice 1 lemon

Crushed black pepper to taste

4 tbsp fromage frais or natural
unsweetened yoghurt

1 tbsp Pernod (optional)

1   Cut off the green fronds from the top of the fennel and put them
    to one side. Thinly slice the first 1cm/½in of each fennel bulb and
    put this to one side. Chop the fennel in half, put it cut side down
    onto a chopping board and roughly cut it into even sized pieces
    about 2cm/1 in square.

2   Sauté the onion in the oil for 2 minutes. Add the fennel and
    potato, sauté for 3 - 4 minutes and then add the stock. Bring to the
    boil, cover, reduce the heat and simmer for 15 - 20 minutes until
    the fennel is tender.

3   Turn the heat to low, add the lemon juice, black pepper and the
    fromage frais or yoghurt and blend until smooth with a hand
    blender.

4   Stir in the salmon and finely sliced pieces of fennel and bring the
    soup slowly to the boil. Simmer it over a low heat for 5 minutes.
    The salmon should be just set. Stir in the Pernod.

5   Finely chop the green fronds of the fennel that you have put to
    one side and scatter them over the soup as a garnish before
    serving.

Cullen Skink

Cullen Skink is a traditional Scottish fish stew with a history that goes back hundreds of years. You do not need to stick rigidly to the recipe as you can make the soup from just about any fish or shellfish that you have available. However, the one thing you do need to include is some smoked fish, preferably fish that has been naturally smoked and not dyed.

SERVES 4
1 large leek
1 medium onion
1 stick of celery very finely sliced
2 tbsp butter
2 tbsp plain flour
600ml/20fl oz (1pt) milk
300ml/10 fl oz (½pt) water
2 large potatoes peeled and cut into small cubes

450g/1lb un-dyed smoked haddock with skin and bones removed
115g/4oz small courgette cut into small dice
225g/8oz white fish with skin and bones removed
225g/8oz salmon with skin and bones removed
16 frozen mussels, shells removed

1   Trim the leek and discard any dark green leaves. Slice the leek and onion thinly.

2   Cut the fish into small 1cm/½in dice.

3   Melt the butter in a large saucepan and fry the leek, onion and celery over a medium heat for about 5 minutes.

4   Still with the pan on a medium heat, stir in the flour and cook it for 2 minutes stirring it occasionally, Be careful not to let it brown. Add the milk and water and stir until the liquid comes to the boil and thickens. If you turn the heat too high the sauce at the bottom of the saucepan will stick and burn.

5   Add the potatoes and bring the soup back to the boil. Reduce the heat to very low and simmer for 15 minutes or until the potatoes

are tender.

6   Increase the heat a little and add the courgettes, the fish and the mussels and bring the soup to the boil. Turn the heat back to low and simmer for 5 – 7 minutes.

7   Season with black pepper and garnish with some finely chopped chives or chopped dill before serving.

BAKES, BURGERS & GRATINS

I am sorry to say that in order to treat gout and inflammation meat is off of the menu, at least in the short term. For most people the thought of 'going vegetarian' does not fill them with enthusiasm. Well 'vegie' food is not as bad as you think .

Vegetables and fruit are simply packed full of goodness and they taste great. They contain vitamins, minerals, trace elements and large amounts of antioxidants. Many have anti-inflammatory properties. Flavonoids and bioflavonoids, phytonutrients, anthocyanins, carotenes, quercetin, resveratrol and polyphenols are just some of a long list of health giving compounds that fruit and vegetables contain. You name it they've got it.

Have you ever wondered why fruit and vegetables are so colourful? Flavonoids and bioflavonoids, their old name was tannins, and lycopene are compounds that give vegetables and fruit, grains, leaves and flowers their colour, colours that range from red and orange to purple, mauve and blue. These compounds protect the plants from ultra violet light, disease and predators. The general rule is the brighter and stronger the colour, the greater the health benefits.

Green leafy vegetables, celery, beans, sweet potatoes, squashes, peppers, aubergines, pumpkins, berries, apples, oranges, lemons and limes. The list of vegetables and fruit that are available for us to eat is massive. We are wired to eat them and whether you eat them raw or cooked, they should form a major part of a diet to treat gout and inflammation. Eating at least five portions of vegetables and fruit a day is good sound advice.

Tomatoes are particularly interesting vegetables as they break all of the rules about cooking. Whereas with most vegetables their nutritional content, especially Vitamin C and other antioxidants, is damaged by cooking, with tomatoes it is not. The intense vibrant colour of a tomato is due to a very powerful antioxidant called lycopene that it contains. Lycopene is the major carotenoid found in red fruit and vegetables. Instead of being damaged or destroyed by cooking lycopene actually becomes more bio-available and this makes tomatoes a very valuable source of antioxidants. Just remember that some people can have an adverse reaction to tomatoes and other members of what is called "the nightshade" family of plants. Aubergines (egg plants), peppers and potatoes are also in this group.

Pulses are a particularly valuable vegetable as they are low in carbohydrate but high in protein, fibre and resistant starch. Red and black beans, chick peas, butter beans, borlotti beans, haricot beans, lentils and dried split peas are the staple food of millions of people around the world.

With only a few exceptions all vegetables are anti-inflammatory but which vegetables are the most anti-inflammatory? Onions, carrots, sweet potatoes, spinach, squashes, pumpkin, kale and sprouted seeds like alfalfa, mustard cress and amaranth. Onions contain some interesting anti-inflammatory chemicals, including the phytonutrient quercertin and the compound allicin, which breaks down to form a powerful antioxidant.

Eat as many vegetables as you want. They are on 'free issue' in an anti-inflammatory diet. Be a bit careful about grapes and apples and other fruits that contain large amounts of fructose. In reality unless you eat your way through a several hundred grams of grapes or an awful lot of apples you are unlikely to be eating enough during a day to cause any real problems in terms of excess fructose consumption.

Eat your vegetables raw as a salad, steamed, braised, baked or stir fried very quickly at not too high a heat, more lightly sautéed than fried. The less you cook them the more nutritious the vegetables are. In reality you cannot eat too many vegetables.

CONTENTS

Aubergine Melanzane

One of the delights of Italian cooking that has found its way around the world. Melanzane benefits from being cooked and then reheated as this allows the flavours develop. It freezes very well. Serve it with a simple green salad or some green vegetables.

SERVES 4

1½ kg/3lbs Aubergine

2 tbsp olive oil (or the oil from the tin of anchovies)

500ml/18fl oz Passata (sieved tomato)

3 tbsp Tomato purée

2 tsp vegetable stock powder

250g/8oz) Mozzarella or Feta

2 - 3 cloves of garlic - crushed

Finely grated parmesan

Large handful of basil leaves

2 tbsp chopped black olives and/or capers

80g Tin anchovy fillets in olive oil

1 Pre heat the oven to 180°C/ 350°F/Gas 4

2 Slice the aubergines about 5mm/¼in thick.. Put them into a microwave bowl, cover and microwave on full power for about 5 minutes until they are soft.

3 Heat the Passata, stir in the tomato concentrate, the bouillon powder, the crushed garlic and the oil. Leave to simmer on a low heat for about 10 minutes.

4 Grease a wide shallow ovenproof dish or tin. Put a layer of the cooked aubergine over the base, then add some tomato sauce, some torn basil leaves, olives or capers, some of the cheese and a scatter of parmesan.. Add another layer of aubergine, tomato sauce, basil, cheese and olives and finish with a layer of tomato.

5 Tear up the anchovy fillets and scatter them over the top. Bake for 45 minutes.

Pumpkin & Roquefort Cheesecake

This recipe came from one of those 'what have I got in the fridge?'
moments. It is not strictly a cheesecake as it uses silken tofu instead of
cream cheese. You can use pumpkin or butternut squash, any type of
blue cheese and you can eat the cheesecake either hot or cold. The
cheesecake does not freeze.

SERVES 6 – 8

350g/12oz packet Silken Tofu

3 large free range eggs

150g/5½oz Roquefort or other
blue cheese

600g/1lb 5oz pumpkin or 1
medium butternut squash

225g/8oz cauliflower broken into
small florets

For the base

60g/2¼oz whole grain spelt OR
buckwheat

60g/2¼oz fine oatmeal

20g/½oz toasted oatmeal

1 tsp baking powder

50g/1¾oz ready made gremolata

1 tsp garlic powder

250ml/9 fl oz milk

The recipe for gremolata is on page 256. Alternatively use 2
tablespoons of finely chopped parsley and a teaspoon of grated
lemon zest. You will need a 24cm/10 in silicon cake tin or spring form
tin with a loose base to make this. If you are using an ordinary tin
grease it well.

Pre heat the oven to 220ºC/ 450ºF/Gas 6

1   There is no need to peel the pumpkin, just cut it into wedges. If
you are using butternut squash, again there is no need to peel it,
just cut it in half lengthways. Lightly oil a large pan or baking tray
and put the pumpkin in a single layer or place the butternut
squash cut side down. Bake the pumpkin for 20 minutes. The
butternut squash will probably need 30 minutes. Take it out of the
oven and leave it to cool.

2   While the pumpkin is cooking make the base. Mix the spelt (or

buckwheat), fine oatmeal, toasted oatmeal, garlic powder and baking powder together. Mix the gremolata into the milk.

3   Add the milk and gremolata mixture to the flour. It will start bubbling as soon as the milk is added to the flour so mix it quickly to form a batter and pour it into the cake tin. Put it into the oven straight away and bake for 12 – 15 minutes. By this time it should be lightly browned and firm to the touch. Leave it in the tin while you prepare the cheese cake mixture.

4   Turn the oven down to 180°C/ 350°F/Gas 4

5   Put the cauliflower into a microwave bowl with a couple of tablespoons of water, cover and cook on full power for 5 minutes. Drain and put to one side.

6   When the pumpkin or butternut squash is cool enough to handled take off the skin and cut it into 2½cm 1in chunks.

7   Take the base out, turn it over and put it back into the tin.

8   Mix the tofu, Roquefort cheese and the eggs together using a hand blender. Stir in the pumpkin (or butternut squash) and the cauliflower, pour it on top of the base, put it in the oven and bake for 15 minutes. Turn the oven down to 160°C/ 325°F/Gas 3 and bake for another 30 minutes. Leave in the tin for at least 15 minutes before serving.

Variation:
For the base, omit the gremolata and add 1 tsp sweet paprika, 1 tsp dried oregano and ½ tsp smoked paprika. For the cheesecake use 200g/7 oz feta or goats cheese instead of the Roquefort and add 16 oven dried tomatoes cut into quarters and some salted black olives with their stones removed.

Carrot, Lentil & Pistachio Loaf

This recipe uses silken tofu to add additional protein to the lentils. The loaf makes a substantial family meal. It can be made in advance, cooked and then warmed up when needed. It does not freeze well once it is cooked but it can be frozen uncooked.

SERVES 4 - 6

1 large free range egg

50g/1½oz finely chopped coriander

OR 30g/1oz coriander pesto

2 tbsp grated ginger

200g/6½oz red lentils

400g/13oz carrots, peeled and finely grated

50g/1½oz shelled pistachio nuts

350g/12oz silken tofu

1 clove garlic crushed (optional)

Grease and line a 1.4Lt/2 ½ pt loaf tin and heat the oven to 180°C/ 350°F/Gas 4

1 Wash the lentils and pick them over carefully to make sure there is no grit in them. Drain them in a sieve, put them into a saucepan and add 350ml/12 fl oz of cold water. Bring them to the boil, cover, turn down the heat to low and cook very slowly for 20 minutes. The lentils should be just cooked and the water absorbed. Leave them to cool a little.

2 Put the grated carrot and the grated ginger into a microwave bowl. Cover and cook on full power for 5 minutes. Take off the cover and leave to cool a little.

3 Drain the tofu and put it into a large bowl with the egg, Use a hand blender to blend it thoroughly into a thick paste.

4 Add the grated carrot, the cooked lentils, the garlic, pistachio nuts and the chopped coriander to the tofu and egg mixture. Give it a good stir and put it into the loaf tin and bake for half an hour. Turn the oven down to 160°C/ 325°F/Gas 3 and bake for another 30 minutes. Leave for 5 to 10 minutes before serving.

Celery & Almond Roast

You can use silken tofu or a low fat cheese like Quark or Ricotta. The roast can be eaten hot or cold. It does not freeze but it will keep in the fridge for 2 to 3 days.

SERVES 4 – 6
350g/12oz silken tofu
500g/1lb 2oz celery finely sliced
100g/3½oz flaked oats
4 tbsp finely grated parmesan
200g/7oz toasted flaked almonds

2 tbsp chopped parsley
½tsp ground turmeric
3 free range eggs
finely grated zest of a lemon
juice of a lemon

Heat the oven to 180°C/ 350°F/Gas 4

1   Put the finely sliced celery into a microwave bowl, cover and cook on full power for 5 minutes. Give it a stir, put the cover back on and cook for another 5 minutes. Leave it to cool slightly.

2   Put the flaked almonds onto a baking tray and bake them for 6 minutes. Just long enough for them to take on some colour.

3   Put the silken tofu into a large bowl, add the eggs, turmeric and lemon zest and give everything a whiz with a hand blender until the tofu is thoroughly amalgamated with the eggs.

4   Stir in the grated parmesan, the flaked oats, parsley, celery, toasted almonds and lemon juice.

5   Grease a 1½Kg/3lb 6oz loaf tin, spoon in the mixture and press it down. Cover with foil and bake for 30 minutes at 180°C/ 350°F/Gas 4.

6   Turn the oven down to 160°C/ 325°F/Gas 3, take off the foil and cook for another 30 minutes. Leave the roast to stand for 10 – 15 minutes before turning it out of the tin.

Mushroom & Chestnut Stuffed Onions

This is an old way of serving onions. In the past the chestnuts would have been roasted on a fire. In the absence of a fire the easiest option is to use ready to use, vacuum packed or frozen chestnuts.

SERVES 4

4 large white onions

200g/7oz chestnut mushrooms finely chopped

200g/7oz packet of ready cooked chestnuts

1 large stick of celery finely chopped

1 tbsp olive oil

1 tsp balsamic vinegar

3 cloves garlic crushed

2 tsp dried rosemary

1 tsp sweet paprika

½ tsp smoked paprika

Zest ½ lemon

Juice ½ lemon

2 tbsp medium or fine polenta

1 Peel the onions. Trim off the bottom so that they stand upright. Cut them in half 'horizontally' and trim the top so that the top half also stands upright.

2 Hollow out the onions leaving 3 rings or layers on the outside. The easiest way to do this is to push the inside onion rings up through from the cut top and bottom. Finely chop the onion you have taken out.

3 Pre heat the oven to 200ºC/ 400ºF/Gas 5

4 Heat the oil over a medium heat and cook the chopped onion, celery, garlic and mushrooms for 10 – 15 minutes until they are tender.

5 Stir in the rosemary, paprika, lemon zest, lemon juice and balsamic vinegar.

6 Roughly chop the chestnuts and stir them into the onion and

mushrooms.

7   Arrange the onion halves in a single layer in a greased oven proof
    dish or casserole. Stuff the onions with the mushroom and
    chestnut mixture and drizzle a small amount of olive oil over each
    one.

8   Add 4 tablespoons of water to the dish, cover and bake for 45 - 60
    minutes until the onions are tender.
    Serve hot from the oven or cover and store in the fridge for a day.

Note:

If you have any of the onion and chestnut stuffing mixture left over
you can make it into pâté Add the juice of the other half of the lemon
and 2 tablespoons of finely grated parmesan. Then blitz it with a hand
blender. You can store the pâté in the fridge for a day or two and it
also freezes well.

Pumpkin, Tomato & Chestnut Bake

You can use pumpkin, butternut squash or sweet potatoes to make this.

SERVES 4

1½ Kg/3lb 6 oz small pumpkin or butternut squash

1 tsp oregano

1 tsp chilli flakes

1 tbsp olive oil

200g/7oz cherry tomatoes

2 balls mozzarella cheese cut into slices

Small handful of basil leaves

12 cooked chestnuts cut into quarters

2 tbsp balsamic vinegar

60g/2¼oz packet baby spinach leaves

1   Pre heat the oven to 200°C/ 400°F/Gas 5

2   Peel the pumpkin or butternut squash, remove the seeds and chop it into large chunks. Put it into a bowl and add the olive oil, oregano and chilli flakes and season to taste.

3   Put the pumpkin or butter squash onto a roasting tray lined with non stick foil and bake for 20 minutes. Turn it over half way through.

4   Add the cherry tomatoes and the chestnuts and turn them over with the pumpkin or squash. Cook for 10 minutes.

5   Stir in the mozzarella and basil leaves and drizzle over the balsamic vinegar before serving on a bed of baby spinach leaves.

Vegetables Baked With Tamarind

A quick and easy way to cook winter vegetables. You can use sweet potato or butternut squash for this recipe and any root vegetables that you have available. Serve them with some green vegetables or piled on top of Socca. A recipe for Socca is in the section on Pasta, Gnocchi and Pizza.

The essential ingredient in this is tamarind. This gives the vegetables a distinctive tart slightly sour flavour. Instructions for making the tamarind pulp are in the section on Herbs and Spices. If you are unable to obtain tamarind use lemon or lime juice instead.

SERVES 4 - 6

1 large butternut squash, peeled, de-seeded and cut into 2cm/1 inch chunks

450g/1 lb cooked beetroot.

16 small new potatoes cut in half

16 small banana shallots peeled

4 small turnips

3 tbsp olive oi3 tbsp tamarind pulp

1 tsp Sambol Oelek or finely chopped red chilli

2 large firm eating apples

3 tbsp lightly toasted pumpkin seeds

1 crushed clove of garlic (optional)

2 tbsp finely chopped parsley or coriander

Pre heat the oven to 200ºC/ 400ºF/Gas 5

1 Blanch the shallots by putting them into a pan of water, bring to the boil and simmer for 3 minutes. Drain.

2 If the beetroot are large cut them into half or quarters. Cut the turnips into quarters. Peel and core the apples and cut each of them into six pieces.

3 Mix half of the tamarind pulp with 2 tbsp of the olive oil,

4 Put a large baking tray lined with non stick foil into the oven to heat for a few minutes.

5 Put all the vegetables into a large bowl, add the oil and tamarind mixture and give the vegetables a good stir to make sure they are well coated. Turn them onto the heated try and bake for 20 minutes until they are tender.

6 Mix the remaining tablespoon of olive oil with the remaining tamarind. Remove the vegetables from the oven and drizzle over the tamarind and oil and pop them back into the oven for another 5 minutes.

7 Pile the vegetables on top of the Socca and sprinkle over the pumpkin seeds and chopped herbs. Serve with a green vegetable and some garlicky natural yoghurt or Tahini

Variation:

A slightly under ripe mango, peeled and cut into chunks can be used instead of the apple.

Spinach & Red Pepper Moussaka

This is a cross between a spinach pie and a Moussaka. Traditionally a spinach pie is cooked in a case of filo pastry and a moussaka is made with a meat stew that is cooked between layers of aubergine. Like most aubergine dishes this moussaka freezes well so you can freeze any leftovers or make it in advance especially for the freezer. If you do freeze it you do not need to complete the final baking process. You can use fresh peppers that you roast yourself or you can use ready roasted peppers that are sold in jars and cans.

SERVES 4

600g/1lb 5oz aubergine plus olive oil for brushing

400g /14 oz cooked spinach or Swiss chard

2 tbsp pine nuts lightly toasted

200g /7 oz feta crumbled

6 spring onions finely sliced

3 large red peppers OR a jar of roasted red peppers

For the béchamel sauce

40g / 1½oz plain flour

500ml / 18 fl oz milk

60g / 2oz grated parmesan

1 egg beaten

Grated nutmeg and ground black pepper.

1   Preheat the oven to 180°C/ 350°F/Gas 4 and Grease a large dish, about 5cm/2 inches deep.

2   Slice the aubergines into rounds 1cm /½ inch thick. Line two baking trays with foil and brush them with oil. Put the sliced aubergines onto the trays and lightly brush them with oil. Bake them at 180°C for 15 minutes. The aubergine should be soft but not brown. Put the cooked aubergine to one side

3   If you are using fresh red peppers, turn the oven up to 200°C/ 400°F/Gas 5. Cut the red peppers in quarters and roast them for 30 minutes until the skin is beginning to blister and look charred. Put them into a dish, cover them with cling film and leave them to cool

a little. Peel the skins off of the peppers and tear them into strips. Reserve any oil that has come out of them.

4   Make the béchamel sauce. Melt the butter on a gentle heat and stir in the flour. Cook gently for a couple of minutes. You do not want the flour to take on any colour.

5   Using a whisk, slowly add the milk and keep whisking. Most recipes tell you to warm the milk when making a sauce to prevent lumps forming. If you use a whisk there is no need to warm the milk. When all the milk is added stir in the grated parmesan and cook gently for 5 minutes, stirring occasionally. Turn off the heat.

6   Squeeze the spinach or chard to make sure it is dry and mix it with the toasted pine nuts, chopped spring onions and the crumbled feta.

7   Pour about a quarter of the béchamel sauce over the bottom of the dish and place a layer of the cooked aubergine on top. Add the spinach mixture and on top of this pour another quarter of the béchamel sauce.

8   Put in another layer of cooked aubergine and then the red peppers. Top the peppers with the remaining aubergine.

9   Beat the egg and mix it with the remaining béchamel sauce and pour this over the top layer of aubergine.

Bake for 45 minutes. Serve with a green salad or some green vegetables.

Layered Parsnip, Nut & Mushroom Roast

This recipe is delicious served either hot or cold. You can use any type of nut to make it. Roasting the nuts for 8 minutes will bring out their flavour.

SERVES 6

225g/8oz chestnut mushrooms
1 tbsp butter
110g/4 oz pecan nuts or walnuts
60g/2oz toasted flaked oats
1 free range egg
450g/1lb peeled and cored parsnips
375g/12oz frozen leaf spinach
½ tsp dried thyme
½ tsp dried rosemary
1 tsp sesame oil

1 tsp garlic granules
250ml/8 fl oz cooking water from the parsnips
1 heaped tsp vegetable stock powder
100g/3½oz feta chopped into small cubes
3 spring onions finely sliced

Set the oven to 180ºC/ 350ºF/Gas 4 and grease a 900g/2 lb loaf tin

1 Put the pecan nuts onto a roasting tray and roast them for precisely 8 minutes. Any longer and the nuts will burn. Take them out of the oven and leave them to cool.

2 When the pecan nuts are cold grind them in a blender or food processor and then mix them with the flaked oats.

3 Cook the frozen spinach following the cooking instructions on the packet and drain really well.

4 Roughly chop the parsnips, put them in a saucepan of cold water, bring them to the boil and cook for 15 minutes until they are tender.

5 Put the vegetable stock powder into a jug and pour on 250ml/ 8 fl oz of the cooking water from the parsnips to make a stock. Then drain the parsnips. Mash them and season with pepper and salt.

6   Melt the butter in a saucepan, slice the mushrooms and sauté them for 5 minutes. Stir in the rosemary and thyme and the sesame oil. Add the cooked spinach and leave to cool slightly.

7   Add the beaten egg and stock to the ground pecan nuts and flaked oats, stir in the sliced spring onions and then add the mashed parsnips. Put half of the parsnip and pecan nut mixture in the bottom of the prepared loaf tin. Press it down well.

8   Mix the feta with the mushroom and spinach mixture and put this on top of the parsnips. Press it down and then add the rest of the parsnip and cashew nut mixture.

9   Cover with foil and bake for 45 minutes. Take the foil off and cook for another 15 minutes.

If you are serving this hot leave it for 10 minutes before turning it out of the loaf tin.

Baked Aubergine with a Walnut Salsa

An essential ingredient in this recipe is walnuts that have been picked before the shells have formed and then pickled. They give the salsa its characteristic flavour. The aubergines can be eaten hot or at room temperature.

SERVES 4

2 large aubergines
2 tbsp olive oil

For the Salsa
85g/ 3oz chopped walnuts or
pecan nuts
60g /2½oz pickled walnuts
chopped into small pieces
85g/ 3oz crumbled feta or goats cheese
1 tbsp pickling liquid from the pickled
walnuts

2 tbsp cider vinegar
1 clove garlic crushed
1 tsp Sambol Oelek or finely chopped
red chilli
2 tsp walnut oil
1 tbsp chopped parsley
2 tbsp chopped coriander
1 tbsp pomegranate seeds OR 1 tsp of
ground dried pomegranate seeds
(optional)
100g/3½oz cooked quinoa (optional)

1   Pre heat the oven to 200°C/ 400°F/Gas 5. Cut the aubergines in half lengthways. Put them onto a baking tray flesh side up and score the flesh in a criss-cross pattern. Brush them with oil, loosely cover with foil and bake for about 30 minutes until the flesh is soft and cooked through. Remove the aubergines from the oven and take off the foil.

2   To make the salsa, mix together the walnuts, the chopped pickled walnuts, the vinegar, oil, pickled walnut liquid, garlic, Sambol Oelek, the chopped parsley and half of the coriander. If you are using it stir in the cooked quinoa.

3   Spoon the salsa over the aubergine flesh. Just before serving add the crumbled feta and the remaining coriander. Lightly sprinkle with the powdered pomegranate seeds.

Mushroom, Buckwheat & Walnut Roast

This is a rich dark bake that can be served either hot or cold. The main ingredients are buckwheat, pecan nuts or walnuts, mushrooms and spinach. You can use fresh spinach but in order to make it quick and simple this recipe uses frozen spinach.

SERVES 4

110g/4oz buckwheat

110g/4oz white onions finely chopped

225g/8oz chestnut mushrooms

110g/4oz walnuts or pecan nuts

8oz frozen leaf spinach

1 tsp dried rosemary

1 tsp dried sage

1 large free range egg

1 tbsp butter or ghee

salt and ground black pepper to taste.

1 Grease a 900g/2lb loaf tin and pre heat the oven to 180°C/ 350°F/Gas 4.

2 Wash the buckwheat in several changes of water. Drain, put it into a saucepan and cover it with water. Bring it to the boil, cover and simmer for 20 minutes. Drain and put to one side.

3 Cook the frozen spinach following the instructions on the packet. Put it into a sieve and drain really well.

4 Heat the butter in a saucepan and sauté the chopped onions for 2 -3 minutes, then add the sliced mushrooms, the rosemary and the sage. Give everything a good stir, put on the lid, turn down the heat and cook for 10 minutes.

5 Grind the walnuts or pecan nuts. Beat the egg. Mix the mushroom and onions with the cooked buckwheat, add the spinach, ground nuts and mix with the beaten egg.

6 Press the mixture into the loaf tin and bake for 50 to 60 minutes. Leave to rest for 10 minutes before removing it from the tin.

Sweet Potatoes with Ginger & Beans
You will need orange sweet potatoes for this recipe.

SERVES 4

2 large sweet potatoes peeled and
sliced into 1cm/½ in thick rounds

12 small pickling onions or banana
shallots

400g/14 oz can black beans drained
and rinsed

2 tbsp balsamic vinegar

2 tbsp grain mustard

1 tbsp olive oil

1 tbsp water

1 tbsp finely grated ginger

1 tbsp runny honey

50g/1½oz baby spinach leaves

Heat the oven to 200ºC/ 400ºF/Gas 5

1   Peel the pickling onions or shallots and put them into a saucepan
of boiling water. Cook them for 2 minutes, drain and when they are
cool enough to handle cut them in half.

2   Put the sliced sweet potato and the onions into a large bowl.

3   Mix the water, olive oil, grain mustard, balsamic vinegar and grated
ginger together and pour this over the sweet potato and onions.
Stir and make sure they are well coated with the mixture.

4   Use a slotted spoon to put the sweet potato and onions onto a
non stick baking tray. Bake uncovered for 20 – 25 minutes until the
sweet potato is soft. Baste with the mustard and ginger mixture
half way through.

5   Warm the black beans in a covered bowl in the microwave for 2 to
3 minutes. Then stir in the baby spinach leaves so that they wilt
slightly. When the sweet potatoes are cooked, put them into a
serving dish, and mix in the black beans and wilted spinach.

Brazil Nut & Mushroom Cutlets

A variation on the vegetarian 'nut cutlet'. This recipe uses Brazil nuts as they are a valuable anti-inflammatory nut but you can use any type of nut to make this. The cutlets freeze well and they can be cooked straight from the freezer if necessary. You will find the recipe for the toasted oatmeal coating in the Grains and Rice section.

MAKES 8

400g/14 oz chestnut mushrooms finely sliced

2 tbsp olive oil

100g/3½oz millet

300ml/10 fl oz water

2 tsp vegetable stock powder

1 tsp smoked garlic granules

½ tsp cayenne pepper

1 tsp dried rosemary

2 banana shallots finely chopped

1 tbsp soy sauce

10g/¼oz dried Porchini mushrooms

100g/3½oz Brazil nuts

30g/1oz toasted sunflower seeds

Toasted flaked oatmeal for coating

1   Heat the olive oil in a saucepan and fry the mushrooms for a minute or two. Add a couple of tablespoons of water, put the lid on the saucepan and cook for 3 minutes over a fairly high heat.

2   Take off the lid and cook the mushrooms until most of the fluid has evaporated. Remove the mushrooms from the saucepan and put them to one side while you cook the millet.

3   Break or cut the Porchini mushrooms into small pieces and put them into the saucepan with the millet. Add the chopped shallot, rosemary, vegetable stock power, cayenne pepper and garlic granules and stir in the water and soy sauce. Bring to the boil, cover, reduce the heat to a gentle simmer and cook for 35 – 40 minutes until the water has been absorbed and the millet is fluffy. Leave it to cool for a while.

4   Put the Brazil nuts and toasted sunflower seeds into a blender or food processor and grind them until they are quite fine. They will become quite oily at this stage. Add a third of the cooked mushrooms to the Brazil nuts in the food processor and blend them for a minute.

5   Put the ground nuts and mushrooms into a bowl and add the rest of the mushrooms with the cooked millet and season to taste with salt and pepper. The mixture should be sticking together quite well. Leave it to cool for an hour or two before making it into cutlets.

6   Put some of the toasted oatmeal coating onto a plate. Flour your hands and take a large heaped tablespoon of the mixture and form it into a cutlet shape about 7cm/3in in diameter. Pushing the mixture into a small ring mould is another way of doing this. Put the burgers onto a tray lined with cling film or non stick foil and put them into the fridge until you are ready to cook them. At this stage you can also freeze them.

7   To cook the cutlets, either oil a large non stick pan and fry them for 5 minutes on each side until a crust forms, or put them into a hot oven on a non stick tray for 10 minutes.

Serve the cutlets with vegetables or salad.

Carrot and Chickpea 'Falafel'

Falafel are pâtés or small burgers that are made from a mixture of cooked chickpeas and chickpeas that have been soaked overnight and then ground. Some people find the ground uncooked chickpeas difficult to digest. This is a sort of 'cheats' falafel that uses tinned chickpeas and cooked quinoa to give the pâtés the slightly grainy texture that comes from the uncooked chickpeas. Traditional falafel are deep fried in oil. This version is cooked in a lightly oiled non stick frying pan or grilled.

MAKES about 36

2 x 400g tins chickpeas drained and rinsed

300g carrots or sweet potato finely grated

2 banana shallots finely chopped

100g/3½oz quinoa

200ml/7 fl oz fl oz water

4 tbsp Tahini

3 tsp ground cumin

50g/1¾oz ready made coriander pesto

1tsp garlic granules (optional)

2 tbsp toasted sesame seeds

Coating

200g/7oz medium or fine polenta

finely grated zest of a lime

small bunch fresh coriander

1   Bring the water to the boil and add the quinoa and ground cumin. Stir, put on a lid, reduce the heat to very low and simmer the quinoa for 25 to 30 minutes. Alternatively cook the quinoa in the microwave following the instructions in the section on Grains and Rice.

2   Mix the grated carrot with the chopped shallot and put it into a microwave bowl. Cover and microwave on full power for 4 minutes. Leave it to cool a little.

3   Put the chickpeas into a blender or food processor with the Tahini and garlic granules and blitz them into a coarse pulp. Add 2 tablespoons of the cooked grated carrot and the coriander pesto

to the chickpeas and whiz again.

4   Tip the chickpea mixture into a bowl, add the toasted sesame seeds and the remaining grated carrots and cooked quinoa and mix it all together thoroughly. At this stage it should be sticking together well.

5   To make the coating, put the polenta, grated lime zest and coriander into a blender or food processor and process until the coriander is amalgamated into the polenta. This mixture will turn light green.

6   Put some of the polenta and coriander dusting onto a plate. Take a heaped teaspoon of the chickpea mixture - about the size of a large walnut - and roll it into a ball. Put it onto the polenta mixture and flatten it into a pate shape. Turn it over and make sure the sides are also coated with the polenta. Put onto a baking tray that is lined with cling film or non stick foil and continue until the chickpea mixture is used up. You should be able to make about 3 dozen small pates.

7   Put the pates into the fridge until you are ready to cook them. At this stage they can also be frozen.

8   To cook the pates, lightly oil a large non stick frying pan and cook the pates on each side until a crust has formed. Serve them with a salad or some green vegetables.

Mexican Bean Burgers

These are quick and easy to make and as they freeze well it is worth making a large batch for the freezer. The recipe for the toasted oatmeal coating is in the Grains and Rice section.

SERVES

200g/7oz finely chopped red onion

200g/7oz red cabbage finely sliced

2 x 400g/14 oz cans red kidney beans, drained and rinsed

175g/6oz firm tofu

2 tbsp olive oil

2 tsp ground cumin

2 tsp smoked paprika

2 tbsp sweet paprika

1 tsp chilli powder

4 tbsp chopped coriander

150g/5½oz cooked millet

Fine polenta or toasted oatmeal coating

1   Heat the oil in a saucepan and fry the red onion and the red cabbage for a few minutes. Keep stirring to prevent the cabbage from sticking. Turn down the heat to low and add the ground cumin, the smoked paprika, the sweet paprika and the chilli power. Give everything a quick stir and then add about 3 tbsp water. Cover the pan and cook for 20 minutes. Stir it occasionally to make sure it is not sticking. Leave the onion and cabbage to cool for about half an hour.

2   Put the tofu with half of the red beans and half of the onion and cabbage mixture into a bowl and blitz them with a hand blender until you have a slightly chunky paste.

3   Add the rest of the red beans, the rest of the onion and cabbage mixture and the chopped coriander. Blend lightly. You want to have the burgers blended enough for everything to stick together. You want some whole beans and pieces of cabbage. You don't want to turn it into a mush. Stir in the cooked millet and leave the mixture to cool for an hour or two before moving on to the next stage.

4   Put some fine polenta or toasted oatmeal coating onto a plate.
    Flour your hands with it, take a large heaped tablespoon of the
    mixture and form it into a burger shapes about 7cm/3in in
    diameter. Put the burgers onto a tray lined with cling film or non
    stick foil and put them into the fridge until you cook them. At this
    stage you can also freeze them.

5   To cook the burgers, oil a large non stick pan and fry them for 5
    minutes on each side until a crust forms. Alternatively, lightly brush
    them with oil, put them onto a non stick baking tray and bake
    them at 200ºC/ 400ºF/Gas 5 for 15 to 20 minutes.

Serve the burgers with a green salad and guacamole. The recipe
for guacamole is on page 268.

Thai Bean Cakes

These are a vegetable version of Thai fish cakes. This recipe uses ready made red Thai curry paste but you can make your own curry paste if you wish. As with the other burgers these freeze really well.

SERVES

2 x 400g/14oz tins borlotti beans

450g/16 oz carrots, peeled and coarsely grated

1 large red pepper

Small bunch finely chopped coriander

Grated zest of a lime

2 tbsp Thai red curry paste

110g/4oz cooked French beans

75g/2½oz coconut powder

1 tbsp grated ginger

150g/5½oz cooked millet

Coating

200g/7oz medium or fine polenta

finely grated zest of a lime

small bunch fresh coriander

1 Cut the red pepper in half, de-seed it and chop into small pieces. Put it with the grated carrots into a microwave bowl, cover and cook on full power for 5 minutes. Leave to cool.

2 Chop the cooked French beans into 5mm/¼ in slices.

3 Drain and rinse the borlotti beans. Put them into a large bowl with the coconut powder, the lime zest, the chopped coriander, the curry paste and the grated ginger. Add more curry paste if you like your food hot and 'spicy'.

4 Blitz the mixture very quickly with a hand blender. Be careful not to turn it into a mush. Stir in the carrot and red pepper. If it looks as though it will not stick together give the mixture another short blend. Now stir in the sliced French beans and the cooked millet and mix well. Leave the mixture in the fridge for an hour or two before shaping it into burgers.

5 To make the coating, put the polenta, grated lime zest and coriander into a blender or food processor and process until the

coriander is amalgamated into the polenta. This mixture will turn light green.

6   Put some of the polenta mixture onto a large plate, drop on a heaped tablespoon of the bean mix which should be fairly firm by now, turn it over in the polenta and form it into a pate/burger shape. Put the burgers onto a tray that has been lined with cling film and either put them into the fridge until you are ready to cook them or put them into the freezer.

7   To cook the bean cakes, dust them again with the polenta mix, and fry them in an oiled non stick pan until crisp on both sides. Alternatively, lightly brush them with oil, put them onto a non stick baking tray and bake them at 200°C/ 400°F/Gas 5 for 15 to 20 minutes.

Serve with a Noodle and vegetable salad.

Brazil Nut & Vegetable Korma

A creamy lightly spiced curry. Like most spiced dishes it benefits from being made in advance so that the flavours can develop.

SERVES 4

50g/1¾oz creamed coconut

2 tbsp olive oil

2 medium onions chopped

2 fresh red or green chillies or

2 tsp chilli paste

1 tsp ground cumin

1 tsp ground turmeric

1 tsp ground coriander

1 clove crushed garlic

125g/4 oz ground Brazil nuts or
cashew nuts

1 small cauliflower broken into florets

250g/8 oz courgettes sliced

125g/4 oz sugar snaps

125g/4 oz cooked peas

4 tbsp fresh chopped coriander

1   Roughly chop the coconut and dissolve it in 450ml/16fl oz of boiling water. Heat the olive oil and fry the onion for 5 minutes, stirring occasionally. Add the chillies, garlic and spices. Stir well and cook for 2 minutes over a medium heat.

2   Stir the ground Brazil nuts into the coconut water and then add this to the onion and spices. Bring it to simmering point, cover and turn the heat to low. You can prepare the recipe to this stage and store it overnight in the fridge.

3   Put some water into a saucepan and bring it to the boil. Add the cauliflower and cook for 3 minutes. Stir in the sugar snaps, bring back to the boil, cover and turn off the heat.

4   While the cauliflower is cooking steam the courgettes in a microwave for 3 minutes.

5   Drain the cauliflower and sugar snaps and add them with the courgettes and cooked peas to the nut, spice and onion mixture. Serve garnished with chopped coriander.

Beans In Red Mole Sauce

This is a taste of Mexico at its best and yes, it really does contain cocoa. Strangely, we first discovered the recipe for the sauce when visiting a chilli farm in of all places the UK. As the sauce freezes well it is worth making a batch for the freezer. If you do decide to freeze it leave out the garlic as this can sometime give rise to a slightly musty flavour.

You can add any type of bean or vegetable to the sauce and it also works well with firm tofu or tempeh and the micro protein Quorn, either as a 'Quorn Mince' or as 'Quorn chunks'.

SERVES 6

For the sauce
2 tbsp olive oil
1 large red onion finely chopped
3 cloves garlic crushed
3 tbsp cocoa powder
1 tsp chilli powder
2 tsp ground cumin
1 tsp smoked paprika
1 tbsp sweet paprika
½ tsp salt
1 tbsp dried oregano
2 x 400g/14oz cans chopped tomatoes

2 red peppers finely sliced or diced
400g/14 oz can red or black beans
400g/14 oz black eyed beans

Avocado Salsa:
4 tbsp finely chopped fresh coriander
1 large avocado
Juice of half a lemon or a whole lime
1 tbsp finely chopped red onion

Natural unsweetened Greek style yoghurt
to serve

1   Reserve a small hand full of the red peppers for a garnish. Heat the olive oil in a large saucepan. Add the onion, garlic and the rest of the red peppers and sauté over a medium heat for 5 to 10 minutes. Do not let the onion or garlic brown.

2   In a small bowl mix together the cocoa powder, chilli, cumin, both types of paprika, salt and oregano. Add this to the onion and pepper mixture, stir well and cook, stirring all the time, for a minute or two to bring out the flavour of the spices.

3 Add the canned tomatoes. Give everything a good stir, bring to the boil, turn down the heat and simmer gently for 10 minutes.

Pre heat the oven to 160ºC/ 325ºF/Gas 3

4 Drain and rinse the beans and add them to the sauce. Bring everything back to the boil, then turn off the heat and transfer the beans and sauce to an oven proof dish or casserole. Cook for 30 – 40 minutes while you prepare the salsa.

5 Cut the avocado in half. Remove the stone using a small spoon, then peel and chop it into small pieces. Stir in the lemon juice and add the finely chopped red onion and the chopped coriander.

Serve the beans garnished with the reserved red peppers and with the natural yoghurt and the avocado salsa in separate bowls.

Potatoes with Saffron & Raisins

Cooking them with saffron and raisins gives potatoes an exotic Middle Eastern taste. This casserole can be eaten as soon as it is made or kept over night in the fridge and re heated the next day.

SERVES 4

3 tbsp olive oil

1 large white onion finely sliced

2 cloves of garlic finely sliced

700g/1 lb 8 oz small salad potatoes cut in half or into 1cm/½ in slices

A large pinch of saffron

½ tsp turmeric

1 red chilli finely chopped or 1 tsp Sambol Oelek

2 sticks celery finely chopped

30g/1 oz raisins

1 tsp vegetable stock powder

3 tbsp chopped coriander

Lightly toasted flaked almonds

Pre heat the oven to 160°C/ 325°F/Gas 3

1   Dissolve the vegetable stock powder in 100ml/3 fl oz of hot water and add the saffron.

2   Give the potatoes a good scrub. You only need to peel them if their skins are damaged.

3   Heat the oil in a large casserole, add the sliced onion and the chopped celery and cook, stirring occasionally for 5 minutes.

4   Stir in the sliced garlic, the chilli, turmeric, raisins, potatoes and the saffron and vegetable stock. Bring to the boil, cover and turn off the heat.

5   Transfer the casserole to the oven. The potatoes will need to cook for between 30 and 45 minutes depending on the variety. Check them after 30 minutes to see if they are soft. When they are cooked garnish them with the chopped coriander and the toasted flaked almonds.

Potato & Tomato Bake

This recipe can be cooked like a casserole in the oven or on top of the stove like a stew. You can eat it as soon as it is cooked or reheat it the next day. As with all potato dishes it will not freeze.

SERVES 4

2 x 400g/14oz cans of chopped tomatoes

700g/1 lb 8 oz waxy potatoes

1 large white or red onion finely sliced

2 tbsp olive oil

½ tsp chilli flakes or 1 tsp Sambol Oelek

1 tsp ground coriander

½ tsp garam masala

6 cloves of garlic cut into quarters

110g/4oz feta

Finely grated zest and juice of a lime

Chopped dill, parsley or coriander to garnish

Heat the oven to 160°C/ 325°F/Gas 3

1   Give the potatoes a good scrub. You only need to peel them if their skins are damaged. Cut them into 1cm.½in slices.

2   Heat the olive oil in a large casserole and fry the onions on a medium heat until they are transparent. Add the chilli, ground coriander, garam masala and garlic and stir well.

3   Add the potatoes and grated lime zest, give everything a good stir, then add the tomatoes.

4   Bring to the boil, cover, turn off the heat and put the casserole into the oven to cook for one hour. By this time the potatoes should be soft.

5   To serve, squeeze over the lime juice, crumble the feta over the top and scatter with the chopped herbs.

Red Hot Broccoli & Tofu

This is a simple Italian way of cooking sprouting and tender stem broccoli. The recipe also works well with cauliflower. The original recipe for this uses 2 dried red chillies that are crushed and crumbled into the broccoli. I find this a bit too hot and spicy. Using chilli powder, Sambol Oelek or some other form of chilli paste allows you to adjust the 'heat' in line with your palate. While it is not strictly authentic serving this with some noodles and tofu makes it into a substantial meal. You can coat the tofu in sesame seeds then fry it over a gentle heat for a few minutes or just stir it, uncoated, into the broccoli and noodles.

SERVES 4

1Kg/2ib white or purple sprouting broccoli or sprouting kale.

2 tsp Sambol Oelek. Or chilli paste

1 large Ramiro pepper de-seeded and finely sliced into rings

1 clove garlic crushed

20 dry salted black olives with stones removed

3 tbsp olive oil

100g/3½oz soba, rice or egg noodles

250g/9oz firm tofu

1 egg beaten (optional)

3 tbsp sesame seeds (optional)

1   Slice the tofu into squares about 1cm/½ in thick. Lay them onto kitchen paper and dry them on both sides.

2   Sprinkle the sesame seeds onto a plate. Dip the pieces of tofu into the beaten egg and then coat them with the sesame seeds.

3   Heat 1 tablespoon of the olive oil in a non stick frying pan. When it is hot add the tofu. Reduce the heat to medium to prevent the sesame seeds from burning and cook for 2 minutes on each side. Take the pan off the heat and put to one side.

4   You will need to cook the noodles in line with the instructions on the packet. Usually this means putting them into boiling water, reducing the heat and then simmering them for between 5 and 7

minutes. Drain them and stir in a tablespoon of the olive oil to prevent them sticking together.

5   Heat 1 tablespoon of the olive oil in a large frying pan or wok. Add the red pepper and cook gently for 5 minutes to extract the flavour from the peppers. Add the garlic and the Sambol Oelek or chilli. Turn the heat to low while you cook the broccoli.

6   Trim off any tough stalks and leaves from the broccoli. If the stems are thick make a shallow cross in them as this will speed up the cooking process. Bring a large pan of water to the boil. Add the broccoli, bring it back to the boil and cook for 2 to 3 minutes until just tender. Turn off the heat and add the cooked noodles. Drain the broccoli and noodles.

7   Increase the heat under the peppers to moderate and add the black olives and the broccoli and noodles. Stir and arrange the cooked tofu on the top.

Tfaya with Chickpeas

Tfaya is a dish of stewed onions that is eaten throughout North Africa and the Middle East. It is usually served as an accompaniment to meat dishes but it works really well with firm tofu, chickpeas and other types of beans. It can be kept in the fridge for a day or two and it freezes really well. Serve the Tfaya with a selection of green vegetables or a salad.

SERVES 4

1Kg/2 lb 4oz white onions finely sliced	125ml/4 fl oz water
50g/1¾oz raisins	2 tsp vegetable stock powder
3 tbsp butter or ghee	Finely grated zest of half a small lemon
1 tsp ground black pepper	juice of 1 lemon
1 tsp ground cinnamon	2 preserved lemons de-seeded and finely
1 tsp ground ginger	chopped
½ tsp turmeric	400g/14oz can chickpeas, drained and
Large pinch saffron strands	rinsed
2 tbsp honey	

The onions in this recipe need long slow cooking so if you have a non stick saucepan this is the time to use it.

1   Put the saffron strands into a cup or jug and add 125ml/4 fl oz boiling water and the vegetable stock powder.

2   Heat the butter in a saucepan over a medium heat and add the onions. Stir them and cook for 5 minutes.

3   Add the pepper, ginger, cinnamon, turmeric, lemon zest and salt. Give everything a good stir and add the saffron stock, raisins and the honey. Bring to the boil, cover, reduce the heat and simmer very slowly for 45 minutes. Check the onions a couple of times to make sure they are not sticking.

4   This is where we move into the 'naughty but nice' stage of this

recipe as the onions now need to be caramelised.

Take the lid off of the saucepan, increase the heat and cook the onions, stirring all the time until most of the fluid has evaporated and some of them begin to look slightly brown. Be careful as you do not want the onions begin to burn. Take them off the heat, add the lemon juice and and preserved lemon and put the lid back on the saucepan.

5 When you are ready to serve the Tfaya put the chickpeas into a microwave bowl, cover and cook following the instructions on the tin. When they are cooked stir them into the onion mixture.

Banana Curry

Strange at it may sound this curry tastes really good. The under ripe bananas provide an excellent source of resistant starch and they are a valuable source of protein.

SERVES 4

4 large under ripe bananas
450g/1lb cooked baby new potatoes
1 large white onion finely sliced
2 tbsp olive oil
2 red or green peppers de-seeded and chopped
2 tsp mustard seeds
½ tsp turmeric

1 tbsp finely grated ginger
3 tbsp tamarind pulp
3 cloves garlic crushed
1 tsp curry powder
70g/2½oz creamed coconut
300ml/10 fl oz (½pt) water
70g/2½oz baby spinach leaves

1   Roughly chop the creamed coconut into small pieces.

2   Heat the oil in a large pan and add the mustard seeds. Stir them around until they begin to pop and then add the sliced onion, garlic and green pepper. Sauté over a medium heat for 10 minutes.

3   Stir in the curry powder, grated ginger and turmeric. Cook for a minute or two and then add the water, tamarind pulp and creamed coconut. Stir until the creamed coconut dissolves.

4   Cut the cooked new potatoes in half.

5   Peel and cut the bananas into 2cm/1 in chunks.

6   Stir the bananas and potatoes into the curry mixture. Simmer for 5 to 10 minutes until the bananas are just beginning to soften and the sauce has thickened slightly. Just before serving add the baby spinach and stir until it has wilted.

Chickpea & Cauliflower Curry with Onion Raita

This is a quick, basic curry sauce that you can use to make any type of curry using vegetables, beans, tofu, fish or seafood. This recipe uses cauliflower and chickpeas. Don't be put off by the long list of ingredients.

SERVES 4

For the curry sauce

400g/14oz tin chopped tomatoes

1 medium white or red onion finely sliced

2 tbsp olive oil

2 tbsp grated ginger

2 cloves of garlic crushed

1 red chilli finely chopped OR 2 tsp Sambol Oelek

2 tsp ground coriander

1 tsp ground cumin

½ tsp ground fenugreek

½ tsp turmeric

2 tbsp natural unsweetened yoghurt

Juice and finely grated zest of a lemon or lime

2 tbsp coriander very finely chopped

1 medium cauliflower

400g/14oz can chick peas drained and rinsed

Red Onion Raita

1 tsp cumin seeds

1 clove garlic crushed

1 small chilli (optional)

1 large red onion

200ml/7 fl oz natural unsweetened yoghurt

2 tbsp finely chopped coriander

1 tbsp lemon juice

1 First make the Raita. Toast the cumin seeds for 1 – 2 minutes in a dry pan over a moderate heat. Be careful not to let them burn. Lightly crush them using a pestle and mortar.

2 Put the yoghurt into a bowl and add the cumin, garlic and chilli if you are using it.

3 Finely chop the red onion and add it to the yoghurt mixture. Then stir in the chopped coriander and the lemon juice. Cover and put the raita into the fridge.

4   Remove the skins from the tomatoes by covering them with boiling water and leaving them to soak for a minute or two. Drop them into cold water and then peel them. The skins should come off quite easily. Roughly chop the tomatoes. As an alternative you can use a can of chopped tomatoes.

5   Heat the oil in a saucepan and sauté the sliced onion for 2 -3 minutes. Add the tomatoes, cook for a couple of minutes and then stir in the cumin, ground coriander, turmeric, chilli, garlic lime or lemon zest and the ginger. Add 150ml/5fl oz water, bring to the boil, turn down the heat and simmer for 10 minutes while you prepare the cauliflower.

6   Take the outer leaves off of the cauliflower and break the florets into small thumb size pieces. Bring a pan of water to the boil and cook the cauliflower for 3 minutes.

7   Drain the cauliflower and add it with the chickpeas to the curry sauce. Stir in 2 tbsp chopped coriander, the yoghurt and lime or lemon juice. Cook for a 4 -5 minutes until the chickpeas are heated through and the cauliflower is tender.

8   Serve the curry with the Raita in a separate bowl..

Sweet and Sour Aubergine

An unusual way of cooking aubergine. Serve this dish on its own, with Socca cut into wedges or with a red bean salad. To cook this you will need a wide, deep pan with a well fitting lid.

SERVES 4

2 medium aubergines weighing about 400g / 14oz

1 tbsp olive oil

250g /8oz sliced white or red onion

2 lemons thinly sliced

2 large red Ramiro peppers deseeded and sliced

1 tbsp dark unrefined sugar

5 tbsp cider or wine vinegar

1 heaped tbsp raisins

1 tbsp butter

1 large clove of garlic crushed

250 ml water

1 Heat the oil in the pan and cover the base with the sliced onion and raisins. Reduce the heat to medium while you slice the aubergine in rounds 1cm/½ inch thick.

2 Put a layer of aubergine on top of the onions side by side. On top of each slice of aubergine put a slice of lemon and some slices of pepper. Repeat the layers of aubergine, lemon and pepper until all the aubergine is used up.

3 Mix the 250ml of water with the sugar, the vinegar and the garlic and pour this over the aubergine.

4 Bring to the boil, cover tightly with foil and a lid, turn down the heat and simmer very gently for about 45 minutes. The aubergine should be just soft. Cook for another 5 to 10 minutes if the aubergine is not soft. Remove from the heat and carefully place the individual slices of aubergine, lemon and pepper onto a large plate. A meat dish is ideal for this.

5 Boil the fluid left in the pan until it is reduced and thickened and then pour it over the slices of aubergine.

Quorn with Ginger, Chilli & Leeks

Quorn is the brand name of a versatile micro protein food which, like tofu, absorbs flavour and keeps a good firm texture when it is cooked. This makes it ideal for stir fries. It is available in most supermarkets. You can use firm tofu or Tempeh as an alternative.

SERVES 4

225g/8oz Quorn chunks

2 tbsp olive oil

1 tsp sesame oil

1 tsp Sambol Oelek or 1 finely chopped red chilli

1 tbsp finely grated ginger

2 tbsp light soy sauce

1tbsp dry sherry or vermouth

3 leeks, white only, finely sliced

1 small Ramiro pepper finely sliced

50ml/5 fl oz vegetable stock

1 tbsp cornflour

1   Mix the grated ginger, Sambol Oelek, soy sauce, sherry and sesame oil together in a bowl. Add the Quorn chunks, stir them around and leave them to marinade for 30 minutes.

2   Strain the Quorn from the marinade but keep the marinade. Add the stock, and the cornflour to the marinade to make a paste.

3   Heat the oil in a wok or large frying pan and sauté the Quorn until it is lightly browned. Remove it and put to one side.

4   Sauté the leeks and Ramiro pepper for 4 – 5 minutes until the leeks are tender. Return the Quorn to the pan together with the marinade and cornflour mixture and stir well until the liquid becomes clear.

Quorn Tangine

You can use Quorn or any other type of protein with this basic Tangine sauce. White fish, prawns and tofu all taste really good. Don't be put off by the long list of ingredients. The Tangine can also be made in advance and re-heated when needed.

SERVES 4

½ tsp cayenne pepper

½ crushed black pepper

1 tsp sweet paprika

1 tsp ground turmeric

1 tsp ground ginger

1 tsp ground cinnamon

2 tbsp olive oil

1 large onion chopped

1 large clove of garlic crushed

350g/12oz Quorn chunks

350g/12oz tin chopped tomatoes

1 tbsp tomato purée

1 tbsp runny honey

50g/1¾oz sultanas or raisins

50g/1¾oz ready to eat apricots cut into halves

300ml/10 fl oz (½pt) vegetable stock

35g/1¼oz lightly toasted flaked almonds

Pre heat the oven to 180°C/ 350°F/Gas 4

1. Mix together the cayenne pepper, black pepper, paprika, turmeric, ginger and cinnamon. Put the Quorn pieces into a bowl and sprinkle over half of the spice mix.. Stir well to coat the Quorn with the spices and marinade for 15 minutes.

2. Fry the onion in the olive oil over a gentle heat for 5 minutes. Stir in the remaining spice mix and cook for another 5 minutes until the onion is soft. Add the crushed garlic just before the end.

3. Stir in the chopped tomatoes, vegetable stock , tomato purée, honey, apricots and raisins. Finally stir in the Quorn pieces. Pour the mixture into a gratin dish and bake for 35 – 40 minutes.

4. Scatter over the toasted almonds and serve with green vegetables.

Carrot with Saffron & Cumin

Carrots are naturally quite sweet and braising them brings out their natural sweetness. You can use any type of carrot but young new season carrots are particularly good. You can serve this dish on its own, with vegetable gnocchi, firm tofu or with cooked chickpeas added at the end. You can also turn it into a delicious soup simply by adding some more water and blending it until it is smooth.

SERVES 4

500g/1lb 2oz carrots peeled

3 tbsp olive oil

1 tsp ground cumin

1 tsp cumin seeds

Generous pinch of saffron

150ml/5 fl oz (¼ pt) water

1 tsp vegetable stock powder

4 large cloves of garlic finely sliced

Finely grated zest of half a lemon plus the juice of half a lemon

Salt and ground black pepper

400g/14oz tin chick peas (optional)

2 tbsp chopped dill to garnish

1   Put the saffron to soak in 2 tbsp hot water while you prepare the carrots. Warm the water and dissolve the vegetable stock in it.

2   If the carrots are small leave them whole. If they are large either cut them into quarters lengthways or cut them across at a diagonal to form oval slices about ½cm/¼ in thick.

3   Heat the oil in a large saucepan and add the ground cumin, cumin seeds and sliced garlic. Stir briefly and then add the carrots, stirring constantly to coat them with the oil and spices.

4   Add the saffron and its soaking liquid, the stock and the lemon zest. Bring to the boil, turn down the heat, cover and simmer for about 15 - 20 minutes until the carrots are tender.

The precise cooking time will depend on the size and age of the carrots. New season carrots will cook more quickly. Stir the carrots every 5 minutes to make sure that they do not stick. When the carrots are tender you should have a fairly thick, slightly sticky sauce.

5   Add the vegetable gnocchi, tofu or the chickpeas if you are using them and heat through.

6   Stir in the lemon juice just before serving and garnish with chopped dill.

Serve with green vegetables and a tablespoon of Tahini mixed with 3 – 4 tablespoons of natural unsweetened yoghurt.

Refried Beans

Like the Red Mole Sauce these are a taste of Mexico. You can serve
refried beans on their own or as an accompaniment to tortillas and
frittatas. They go really well with the cheats calzone.

SERVES 4

400g/14 oz can red or black beans
drained and rinsed
1 medium white onion finely sliced
2 tbsp olive oil
2 cloves garlic crushed
1 tsp chilli powder
½ tsp smoked paprika

1 tsp ground cumin
Finely grated zest and juice of a lime
150ml/5 fl oz (¼ pt) water
2 tbsp chopped coriander

1 Heat the oil in a saucepan, add the sliced onion and sauté for 5
   minutes. Stir in the crushed garlic, chilli power, smoked paprika and
   ground cumin.

2 Sauté for 2 to 3 minutes, then add the beans, lime zest and the
   water. Bring to the boil, cover, reduce the heat and simmer for 15
   minutes.

3 Just before serving stir in the lime juice and blend briefly with a
   hand blender to break down some of the beans.

   Serve with fromage frais, natural yoghurt or guacamole.

Sweet & Sour Carrots With Tofu

Use firm tofu to make this dish. You can either braise the tofu in the sauce after the vegetables are cooked, dip it in flour and grill it or fry it in a non stick pan.

SERVES 4 – 6

1½ tsp cornflour

3 tbsp water

175ml/6fl oz vegetable stock

3 tbsp white vinegar

1 tbsp dark unrefined sugar

1 tbsp tomato purée

2 tbsp thin soy sauce

½ tsp cayenne pepper

1 tbsp olive oil

1 clove garlic crushed

2 tbsp finely grated ginger

1 medium white onion peeled and cut vertically into thin crescent shaped wedges

1 medium red pepper chopped into 1cm/½ in squares

1 large carrot peeled and cut into 5mm/¼ in slices

3 spring onions finely sliced

350g/12oz firm tofu cut into 2½cm/1 in cubes

2 tbsp olive oil

2 tbsp roasted cashew nuts roughly chopped (optional)

1 Mix the cornflour with the water in a cup. Combine the vegetable stock, vinegar, sugar, tomato purée, soy sauce and cayenne pepper.

2 Heat 1 tbsp of oil in a saucepan or deep frying pan and sauté the onion, carrot, red pepper and garlic for 3 - 4 minutes. Add the stock and vinegar mixture, bring to the boil, reduce the heat, cover and simmer for 15 minutes until the carrots are tender.

3 Strain the vegetables but reserve the cooking liquid. Put the vegetables into a wide shallow serving dish and keep them warm.

4 Put the stock back into the saucepan and add the cornflour and water mixture. Slowly bring it to the boil and stir until it becomes transparent. Add the tofu, cover, reduce the heat and simmer gently for 5 minutes to cook the tofu through.

5   Carefully place the tofu on top of the cooked vegetables and pour
    over the sauce. Garnish with finely sliced spring onions and
    chopped cashew nuts.

6   If you are frying the tofu, cook it over a medium heat in 1 tbsp
    olive oil for about 5 minutes, turning once. Drain on paper before
    adding to the carrots.

FISH & SEAFOOD

Fish contains large amounts of fatty acids and these, especially the Omega-3 essential fatty acids, have powerful anti-inflammatory properties. Fish is also an excellent sources of protein and other vital nutrients including antioxidants. Cold water oily fish like salmon, sardines, herring, mackerel, trout, and halibut are all excellent sources of Omega-3 but all fish, including shellfish and seafood are a good choice as part of an anti-inflammatory diet. Substitute fish for meat in your diet and try to eat it between two and four times a week.

Unless you live near the coast or have access to a good fishmonger, fresh fish is not easy to obtain. Trout and salmon can usually be found but other than this you will probably have to buy frozen fish. When you do, make sure you thaw it slowly and then wash and dry it thoroughly in order to remove any oils that have oxidised. Unfortunately oily fish like sardines, herring and mackerel do not freeze well so you may have to resort to tins. Just make sure the fish is tinned in water or olive oil and not sunflower or rape seed oil. One way the northern Europeans preserve their oily fish, especially herring, is to pickle it. Bismark herrings and roll mops are usually sold in jars and as they require no cooking they are quick and easy to prepare. Despite the fact that they are salted and then preserved in vinegar that is sometimes sweetened, this type of fish is a very valuable source of healthy oils.

The only downside to fish is that levels of mercury can sometimes be high and this is of some concern. Farmed fish also contains less Omega-3 oils than wild fish. But when you compare the 1,100mg of Omega-3 a 125 gram portion of oily fish contains to the 35mg found in the same amount of lean grass fed beef, eating fish looks quite a good option.

CONTENTS

Herring With Beetroot & Horseradish

This is one of those almost instant meals especially if you have some quinoa already cooked in the freezer. You can use Bismark Herrings or Roll mops to make this recipe. These are ready to eat and usually sold in jars or plastic tubs. The herrings need to be stored in the fridge but as they have a fairly long shelf life they are a useful store cupboard ingredient. All you need to do is drain them before using them in the recipe.

SERVES 4

Large jar 500g/1lb 2oz of Bismarck Herring or Roll mops

100g/3½oz quinoa

230ml/8 fl oz water

500g/1lb 2oz packet of cooked beetroot

Half a medium red onion finely chopped

1 telegraph cucumber

3 – 4 heaped tsp grated horseradish

Juice of a lemon

1 tbsp olive oil (optional)

50g/1¾oz packet baby salad leaves, baby spinach or rocket

To Serve

4 tbsp fromage frais

1 tbsp finely chopped fresh dill

1 tbsp finely chopped capers

1   Quinoa is not the easiest of grains to cook as it needs long, very slow cooking. The easiest way to cook it is by using the absorption method. 100G/3½ oz of quinoa will need approximately 230ml/8 fl oz of water.

2   Wash the quinoa and drain it. Put it into a saucepan, bring it to the boil, cover and reduce to a very, very low heat. Leave it to cook for 25 – 30 minutes. When it has finished cooking leave it to stand for at least a quarter of an hour before taking the lid off. Alternatively cook the Quinoa in the microwave following the instructions in the Grains and Rice section.

3   Leave the Quinoa to cool while you prepare the rest of the
    ingredients.

4   Mix the horseradish with the lemon juice and if you are using it,
    the olive oil in a jam jar. Put on the lid and give it a good shake.

5   Peel the cucumber, cut it in half lengthways and remove the seeds.
    Chop it into small 5mm/¼ in dice.

6   Rinse and dry the beetroot and cut it into small 5mm/¼ in dice.
    Stir the chopped red onion, cucumber, horseradish and lemon juice
    into the Quinoa.

7   Cut the Herrings into bite size pieces and either place them on top
    or mix them with the beetroot and quinoa. You can keep this salad
    in the fridge for up to 24 hours.

8   Mix the fromage frais with the chopped dill and capers and serve it
    in a separate bowl. Serve the Quinoa and herrings on a bed of
    salad leaves or rocket.

Nordic Salad

*There are many different ways of serving oily fish like herrings,
mackerel and sardines that have been preserved. This recipe uses cold
potatoes but you could use cannellini beans as an alternative.*

SERVES 4

Large 500g/1lb 2oz jar Bismark Herring or Roll mops

1 small red onion finely sliced

700g/1 lb 9oz cooked waxy salad potatoes

100g/3½ oz small pickled gherkins

250g/9oz cooked sweetcorn kernels

Hand full of parsley, chervil or dill finely chopped

Baby salad leaves to serve

1   Either slice the cooked potatoes or cut them into 1cm/½ in dice.

2   Slice the gherkins into thin rounds.

3   Wash and drain the sweetcorn.

4   Put the potatoes and gherkins into a large serving dish and add the sweetcorn kernels and the sliced onion.

5   Cut the Bismark Herrings or Roll mops into bite size pieces and place them on top.

6   Garnish with the chopped herbs and serve on a bed of baby salad leaves.

Classic Herrings in Oatmeal

If you are lucky enough to be able to buy fresh oily fish this is a quick and easy way to cook them. You can use herring, sardines, mackerel or trout and you can either fry, grill or bake the fish. In this recipe the fish is baked in the oven.

If you are using herring, mackerel or trout you will need fish that weigh about 300g/10½ oz each when whole. If you are using sardines you will probably need 2 per person. You will find the recipe for toasted oatmeal coating in the Grains and Rice section.

SERVES 2

2 herring, mackerel or trout or 4 sardines	1 tbsp finely chopped capers
About 85g/3 oz toasted oatmeal coating	70g/2½ oz ready made beetroot pesto
2 tbsp flour for dusting	1 clove garlic (optional)
1 large free range egg	

1   Mackerel and trout do not have any scales but if you are using herrings or sardines get the fishmonger to scale the fish as well as clean them. The fishmonger may also bone them but if you have to bone the fish yourself this is what you do.

2   Using a really sharp knife cut along the belly of the fish right down to the tail. Put the fish flesh side down onto a chopping board and use your hand to push down firmly to flatten it out. Then press very firmly along the back bone. This will loosen the backbone and the small bones that are attached to it.

3   Turn the fish over, skin side down, and gently ease the back bone away. Most of the small fine bones will come away with it. Cut the back bone off just above the tail and trim around the belly to tidy the fish up. Use a piece of kitchen paper to wipe off any blood from the fish.

Pre heat the oven to 200°C/ 400°F/Gas 5

4   Put the toasted oatmeal coating into a blender and give it a quick whiz to break it down into smaller pieces.

5   Break the egg into a wide shallow bowl and beat it.

6   You will need a baking tray that is large enough to lay the fish in a single layer. If the tray is non stick lightly bush it with oil otherwise line the tray with oiled baking foil. When the oven is hot put the tray in to get warm.

7   Dust both sides of the fish with seasoned flour, then dip the flesh side only in the beaten egg and then the oatmeal coating, pressing it down firmly. Lightly brush with some olive oil. Put to one side while you process the other fish.

8   Take the baking tray out of the oven and put the fish onto it oatmeal side down. Bake for 10 minutes. Take them out of the oven, turn them over and bake for another 5 minutes.

9   Add the chopped capers to the beetroot pesto and serve this with the fish as soon as they are cooked.

Red Peppers Stuffed with Mackerel

Many vegetables lend themselves to being stuffed and the ingredients you use for the stuffing can be quite versatile. This recipe has its origins in Spain where cooked salt cod is mixed with mashed potato and used to stuff roasted red peppers. Traditionally this is served with a shellfish bisque and it tastes delicious.

This a simple recipe that can be prepared very quickly. You can use any type of fresh or canned fish. The fish used in this recipe is a 'No Drain' can of mackerel fillets that have no added oil. This type of fish is a useful store cupboard ingredient.

SERVES 2

2 large red bell peppers	1 heaped tsp dried dill
1 large potato weighing about 350g/12oz	2 - 3 spring onions finely sliced
110g/4oz tin 'no drain' mackerel fillets	50g/1¾oz prawns (optional)
	1 tbsp Thai fish sauce
1tsp chilli paste or Sambol Oelek	

Pre heat the oven to 180°C/ 350°F/Gas 4

1 Prick the potato and cook it in a microwave on full power for 5 minutes. Turn it over and cook for another 3 -4 minutes until it is just soft.

2 As soon as the potato is cool enough to handle peel off the skin and either mash it or put it through a potato ricer.

3 Cut the peppers in half lengthways through the stem. Remove the seeds and any white pith.

4 Put the peppers cut side up into a lightly greased oven proof pan. You may need to trim the round side a little so that they sit flat. If you end up with a hole put the piece you trimmed off back inside to fill the gap.

5   Break the mackerel fillets into smallish chunks and mix them with the prawns, dill, spring onions, Sambol Oelek and Thai fish sauce into the mashed potato. Divide the mixture between the halved peppers and press it down well.

6   Bake the peppers uncovered for 20 - 25 minutes or until they feel soft when tested with a sharp knife.

Not Quite An Arnold Bennett Omelette

Traditionally an Arnold Bennett omelette is an omelette for 2 people that is topped with smoked haddock and a creamy béchamel sauce.

This is a more substantial version that uses salmon or trout and courgette to turn the omelette into a meal for 4 people. You can use any cut of salmon or trout to make this.

SERVES 4

2 courgettes weighing about 400g/14oz

1 tsp dried dill

6 large free range eggs

1 tsp olive oil

350g/12oz skinned and boned salmon

300ml/10 fl oz (½pt) natural Greek style unsweetened yoghurt

1 tsp cornflour

50g/1¾oz finely grated parmesan or other hard cheese

Salt and pepper to taste

You will need a 26cm/10 in non stick frying pan or chefs pan with a lid to make this.

Pre heat the oven to 200ºC/ 400ºF/Gas 5

1   Wash and dry the salmon and cut it into 1cm/½ in pieces.

2   Whisk one of the eggs, 1 tsp dried dill and 1 tsp cornflour into the yoghurt and put to one side.

3   Whisk the other 5 eggs in a large bowl and season to taste with salt and pepper.

4   Coarsely grate the courgette and mix it into the eggs.

5   Heat the frying pan with 1 tsp olive oil over a medium heat and add the pieces of salmon. Cover and cook them for 5 minutes. By this time the fish should be just set and translucent. Use a slotted spoon to remove it from the pan and put it to one side.

6   Add the egg and courgette mixture to the pan and cook for 5
    minutes over a moderate heat. Put on the lid and transfer the pan
    to the oven. Cook for 10 minutes.

7   Reduce the oven to 180°C/ 350°F/Gas 4

8   Take the frying pan out of the oven, remove the lid and put the
    salmon on top of the 'omelette' in a single layer. Pour the yoghurt
    and egg mixture on top. Put the pan back in the oven without the
    lid and bake for 10 minutes.

9   Pre heat the grill to high. Take the frying pan out of the oven,
    sprinkle on the grated cheese and pop it under the grill until the
    cheese has melted.

    Serve with green vegetables or a green salad.

Salmon Pudding

An easy recipe that uses odd cuts of salmon. You can replace the
courgettes with two finely sliced bulbs of fennel.

SERVES 3 - 4

350g/12oz salmon pieces

1 tbsp olive oil

1 large courgette weighing 200g/7oz

1 large leek, dark leaves removed

6 tbsp natural unsweetened yoghurt

1 tsp dried dill

1 tbsp Thai fish sauce

1 free range egg beaten

For the topping

3 tbsp toasted flaked oatmeal

1 tbsp ready made gremolata OR rocket
pesto

1 tbsp olive oil

1 tbsp finely grated parmesan

1 tbsp capers

Pre heat the oven to 180°C/ 350°F/Gas 4

1   Slice the leek into thin slices. Put it into a microwave bowl with the
    dried dill and 1 tbsp water, cover and microwave on full power for
    5 minutes. Leave it to cool.

2   Top and tail the courgette, cut it into quarters lengthways and then
    cut each quarter into pieces 1cm/½ in long. Put it into a
    microwave bowl with 1 tbsp water, cover and microwave on full
    power for 4 minutes. Drain and leave it to cool.

3   Mix together the toasted oatmeal, pesto, olive oil, grated parmesan
    and capers.

4   Cut the salmon into small even size pieces. Stir the yoghurt, beaten
    egg and Thai fish sauce into the leeks and then add the courgettes.
    Stir in the salmon.

5   Heat the olive oil over a medium heat in an ovenproof casserole
    or chefs pan. Add the courgette, leek and salmon. Sprinkle on the
    oatmeal and pesto mixture and bake for 20 minutes.

Coconut Stuffed Trout

You can prepare this dish in advance and leave it in the fridge until you are ready to cook it. You can either steam the trout, cook it in the microwave or wrap it up in foil and bake it in the oven.

You will need fillets of trout that have been skinned to make this. If you don't have any fresh coconut you can either use grated creamed coconut or soak some dessicated coconut in boiling water for 15 minutes.

SERVES 2

For the stuffing
2 spring onions finely chopped
2 cloves of garlic crushed
Finely grated zest of a lime
Juice of a lime
2 rounded tsp grated ginger
1 tbsp grated coconut
1 tbsp finely chopped coriander

4 skinless trout fillets
8 large lettuce leaves from a soft
round butter head lettuce

1   If the trout has not been skinned you need a chopping board and a very sharp knife.

    Put the fish skin side down. At the tail end of the fillet make a shallow cut that goes down to the skin but not through it. Angle the knife so that the sharp side is facing away from you and cut a little bit of flesh away from the skin. Hold on to the piece of skin and then, with the knife still held at an angle, push lightly at the skin and cut along it to remove the flesh. The skin is quite tough compared to the flesh so the knife should more or less slide over it.

2   Heat the oil and sauté the garlic and spring onions for 2 minutes to cook them a little. Add the lime zest and lime juice, coriander and ginger.

3   Lay the trout fillets skinned side up and divide the stuffing
    between them. Spread it across the fillet and roll the fillet up.

4   To make the lettuce leaves flexible put them into a large bowl and
    pour boiling water over them. Lift them out straight away with a
    slotted spoon and dry them in kitchen paper. Use 2 of these wilted
    leaves to wrap each trout fillet into a parcel.

5   You can use either a bamboo steamer or one of the metal fan
    shaped steamers that adjust to fit the size of the saucepan you are
    using.

6   Put a pan of water on to boil. Put the trout into the steamer in a
    single layer and steam for 10 minutes until the flesh of the trout is
    just set.

Cooking a Whole Salmon

Some cooked salmon or trout in the freezer is a useful store cupboard ingredient, so it is worthwhile cooking a whole salmon or a large piece of salmon and freezing it in portions. These days, as most of us do not own a fish kettle, the easiest way to cook a whole salmon is in the oven, wrapped in foil, provided of course that it will fit into your oven. All you need to do before cooking the fish is to have the salmon cleaned and its scales removed.

1 whole salmon weighing about 1.8Kg/4 lb	3 – 4 fresh bay leaves
1 tbsp olive oil	½ lemon finely sliced
1 small white onion very finely sliced	A handful of parsley, chervil or dill
	½ - 1 tsp crushed black pepper.

The slower the salmon is cooked the better the flavour. Pre heat the oven to 150ºC/ 300ºF/Gas 2

1   There is no need to wash the fish, just wipe it, inside and out, with some kitchen paper. Lay two large pieces of foil, one on top of the other and brush lightly with oil. Lay the fish on the foil and put the sliced onion, bay leaves, sliced lemon and herbs in the cavity. Fold the foil over the fish to make a loose parcel. Fold over the edges of the foil twice to seal it.

2   Place the parcel on a large baking sheet and bake the fish in the centre of the oven for 2½ hours. Remove it from the oven and leave it to cool in the foil.

3   The skin should come off easily when the salmon is cooked and the fish should lift easily from the bones. If you are going to freeze the salmon portion it up, wrap it tightly in cling film and open freeze it in a single layer on a tray before putting it into a box or bag.

Salmon Cured With Dill

Gravlax is an age old way of curing and preserving salmon. It is sold in supermarkets and it is usually quite expensive. However, making your own Gravlax is surprisingly easy. Once cured the salmon keeps in the fridge for up to a week and you can also freeze it.

When you look at the recipe and see the amount of sugar and salt that it uses it doesn't look a healthy option, but the sugar and salt are there only to extract the fluid from the salmon. Once the curing process has finished very little of it will be left in the fish.

You will need a large piece of salmon from the middle of the fish. The salmon needs to be scaled, boned and then pin boned. Classically a Gravlax of salmon should weight about 1¼Kg/2lb 13oz but you can cure any size piece of fish. If the piece of fish you have is larger or smaller just scale the ingredients up or down so that the ratio of sugar and salt to fish is about the same.

SERVES 6 - 8

1¼Kg/2lb 13oz fresh or previously
frozen salmon
3 heaped tbsp dried dill
100g/3½oz sea salt crystals

85g/3oz sugar
2 tbsp crushed black or white peppercorns

You will need a container with a close fitting lid that is large enough to hold the salmon laid flat on its side.

1. If you are using frozen salmon leave it to thaw out over night. Wash it thoroughly and dry it with kitchen paper to remove any oil that may have gone rancid.

   If you are using fresh salmon, wipe it inside and out with damp kitchen paper and remove any blood from the inside.

2. Put the sugar, salt and crushed black pepper into a bowl and mix it together.

3. Put one side of the salmon into the container, spread the salt and sugar mixture over it and sprinkle on the dried dill. Put the other side of salmon on top. All you need to do now is put the lid on the container and then put the container into the fridge.

4. The salmon needs to be turned over twice a day and left to cure for 2 - 3 days depending on the thickness of the fish. As the salmon cures fluid will be drawn out of it and when you turn the salmon over baste the top and inside of the fish with this fluid.

5. When the salmon has cured all you need to do is lift it from the cure, optionally wipe off the dill from the inside and slice it as thinly as possible.

Serve the Gravlax with beetroot pesto, pea sprouts, a green salad or a potato and walnut salad.

Salmon With Cucumber & Potato Salsa

*You can use salmon or trout for this recipe. The fish can be served hot
or cold, either as a fillet or broken into bite size pieces. The cucumber
and potato salsa will keep in the fridge for 2 days.*

SERVES 4

4 fillets of salmon each weighing about
150g/5½oz
½ lemon thinly sliced
4 bay leaves.

For the Salsa:
16 - 20 small cooked new potatoes
1 large telegraph cucumber, peeled,
cut in half lengthways and de-seeded
8 spring onions finely chopped
1 finely chopped green chilli

1 - 2 cloves of garlic crushed
2 tbsp capers drained and roughly chopped
1 tbsp finely chopped fresh dill
1 tbsp chopped flat leaf parsley or chervil
Finely grated zest of 2 limes
Juice of 2 limes
2 tbsp olive oil
Sprigs of fresh dill or parsley to garnish.

Pre heat the oven to 200°C/ 400°F/Gas 5

1   Line a small baking try with foil. Put the fillets of salmon on the foil,
skin side down and tuck a bay leaf under each one. Arrange the
slices of lemon on top of the fish and cover with a piece of foil.
Turn over all 4 edges to seal the fish in a large parcel.

2   Bake the fish for 20 minutes until it is set and translucent. The
precise time it takes will depend on the thickness of the fish. When
the fish is cooked take it out of the oven but leave it in the foil to
rest while you prepare the salsa.

3   Cut the potatoes and cucumber into small 5mm/¼ in dice and put
them into a large bowl. Add the spring onions, chilli, garlic, capers,
dill, parsley and lime zest and give everything a good stir.

4   Put the lime juice and olive oil into a small jar, put on the lid and

give it a good shake. Mix this into the potato and cucumber.

5   When you are ready to serve the fish, put a small pile of the salsa onto a plate and place the fillet of fish on top. Garnish with the herbs. Alternatively you can break the fish into large bite size flakes.

Salmon with Ginger, Lime & Noodles

This recipe works with white fish such as cod, haddock and tilapia as well as salmon and trout. If you do not have any fresh coriander use some ready made coriander pesto from the freezer.

SERVES 2

2 fillets of salmon each weighing about 150g/5½oz
1 tsp grated ginger
Finely grated zest and juice of lime
1 clove garlic crushed

1 tbsp chopped fresh coriander
1 spring onion finely sliced
50g/1¾oz rice vermicelli

Pre heat the oven to 200°C/ 400°F/Gas 5.

1   Soak the rice vermicelli in boiling water for 5 minutes. Drain and refresh in cold water.

2   Remove the skin from the salmon.

3   Mix together the ginger, lime zest, garlic, chopped coriander, spring onion and lime juice.

4   Divide the rice vermicelli between 2 large pieces of non stick foil. Put a fillet of salmon on top. Divide the ginger, lime and spring onion mixture between the fish. Fold over the foil to make a parcel and bake for 20 minutes.

Leave to rest for 5 minutes before serving.

Niçoise Salad

A classic way of serving fresh, frozen or tinned tuna and transforming a small amount of fish into a substantial meal. You can vary both the amount and type of vegetables you use depending on what you have available. If you use frozen tuna try to buy yellow fin tuna steaks that are vacuum packed in individual bags. These are less oxidised and have a much better flavour than the ordinary 'dark' tuna. Don't be put off by the long list of ingredients. This is a very easy recipe to make.

SERVES 4

350g/12oz cherry tomatoes cut in half

110g/4 oz rocket or baby salad leaves

½ telegraph cucumber

175g/6oz fine French beans

450g/1lb cooked small new potatoes OR 400g/14oz can cannellini beans drained and rinsed

8 spring onions sliced

3 - 4 large free range eggs that have been hard boiled

1 tbsp finely chopped flat leaf parsley

20 salted black olives with their stones removed

400g/14oz tin 'no drain' tuna steak OR 4 x small pieces of frozen tuna

For the dressing:

Cooking fluid from the tuna

½ clove garlic crushed

1 tbsp seeded mustard

2 tbsp finely grated parmesan

1 tbsp lemon juice

1 heaped tsp anchovy paste

1   If you are using frozen tuna defrost it slowly at room temperature and then wash and dry it in kitchen paper. Cut each tuna steak in half horizontally into thin pieces.

2   Mix 1 tbsp olive oil with 2 tbsp lemon juice and put it into a saucepan. Bring it to a gentle simmer and then add the pieces of tuna. Bring it back to simmering point, cover and cook for 3 minutes. Turn the slices of tune over and cook them for another 2

minutes. Take if off the heat and leave the tuna to cool while you prepare the salad.

3   Put the French beans into a pan of boiling water. Bring them to the boil and cook them for 3 minutes. Drain them, refresh them in cold water, drain them again and put them to one side.

4   Cut the cucumber in half lengthways and remove the seeds. Cut each half of the cucumber into thin crescent shaped slices.

5   Peel the hard boiled eggs and cut them into quarters.

6   Slice the cooked new potatoes into thin slices.

7   Put the French beans, tomatoes, sliced cucumber, potatoes, olives and spring onions into a bowl and mix well.

8   To make the dressing drain the cooking liquid from the tuna into a jar and mix it with the anchovy paste, crushed garlic, seeded mustard, parmesan and lemon juice. Give it a really good shake to combine the ingredients.

9   When you are ready to serve the salad mix the rocket with the other ingredients and arrange it on a serving plate. Put the pieces of tuna on top and arrange the hard boiled eggs around the edge. Sprinkle on the chopped parsley, Serve the dressing in a separate bowl.

Tuna & Borlotti Bean Salad

This is a famous dish from Tuscany that is one of those 'instant' out of the store cupboard meals. You will need good quality tuna, preferably a 'no drain' brand as you do not want the salad swimming in brine or oil.

SERVES 2 - 4

400g/14oz borlotti or cannellini beans drained and rinsed
120g/4¼ oz can 'no drain' tuna steak in spring water
3 spring onions cut into match stick size slices
Salt and pepper to taste

2 tbsp lemon juice
2 tbsp olive oil
1 tbsp finely chopped parsley or chervil.
50g/1¾oz cooked fine French Beans (optional)
30g/1oz baby spinach leaves

1 Put the olive oil and lemon juice together in a jar and give it a good shake.

2 Mix the borlotti beans, spring onions and, if you using them, the French Beans together in a bowl and stir in the dressing.

3 Break the tuna into small pieces and arrange them on top of the beans. Scatter the parsley or chervil on top and serve on a bed of baby spinach leaves.

Creole Tuna Salad

This tuna salad is far removed from the more usual 'tuna, sweetcorn and mayonnaise' salad. It is one of those salads that you can make from more or less any ingredients that you have available and it is most definitely more salad than fish. As with the borlotti bean and tuna salad you need good quality 'no drain' tuna steak.

SERVES 2 – 4

1 large carrot coarsely grated
1 red pepper finely chopped
½ small red onion finely chopped
1 small green under ripe mango
1 green chilli finely chopped OR
1 tsp Sambol Oelek or chilli paste
50g/1¾oz finely shredded
cabbage or Chinese leaf

120g/4¼ oz can 'no drain' tuna steak in spring water
Finely grated zest and juice of a lime
2 tbsp chopped coriander or what ever herbs you have available
2 tbsp lightly toasted pumpkin and sunflower seeds

1   Remove the stone from the mango. Peel it and cut it into 1cm/½ in chunks. Put it into a large bowl and stir in the lime zest, lime juice and chopped chilli.

2   Add the grated carrot, red pepper, chopped onion and shredded cabbage.

3   Break up the tuna on a plate and stir it in. Garnish with the chopped herbs and toasted seeds.

Serve with green or red Tabasco or hot pepper sauce.

Red Peppers Stuffed with Fish & Leeks

Stuffed peppers are quick and easy to prepare. You can use any type of fresh white fish for this recipe.

SERVES 2

2 large red peppers	5 tbsp natural unsweetened yoghurt
1 large leek about 250g/9oz	1 tsp dried dill
1 large free range egg	1 tbsp Thai fish sauce
225g/8oz white fish	

Pre heat the oven to 180°C/ 350°F/Gas 4

1   Finely slice the leek, put it into a micro wave bowl, cover and cook on full power for 5 minutes. By this time the leek should be soft. Put it to one side to cool a little.

2   Cut the peppers in half lengthways through the stem. Remove the seeds and any white pith.

3   Put the peppers cut side up into a lightly greased oven proof pan or baking tray. You may need to trim the round side at the bottom a little so that they sit flat. If you end up with a hole put the piece you trimmed off back inside to fill the gap.

4   Wash and dry the fish and cut it into small pieces about 1cm/½ in square. Beat the egg and dried dill into the yoghurt and stir it into the cooked leeks. Add the Thai fish sauce and the fish and mix well. Divide the mixture between the halved peppers.

5   Bake the peppers uncovered for 20 minutes or until they feel soft when tested with a sharp knife

Tilapia in Tomato & Cardamom Sauce

This recipe originates from the Middle East. It is a basic tomato sauce that can be used with any type of white fish or shellfish. If you leave out the garlic you can make a large batch of the sauce and store it in the freezer. Adjust the amount of chilli or Sambol Oelek you use to suit your taste.

SERVES 4

400g/14oz can chopped tomatoes

3 tbsp tomato purée

1 medium white or red onion chopped

1 tbsp olive oil

3 cloves garlic crushed

1 chopped chilli or 1 tsp Sambol Oelek

4 tbsp chopped fresh dill OR 2 tsp dried dill

2 tsp ground cumin

1 tsp ground cardamom

Ground black pepper to taste

4x fillets Tilapia weighing about 150g/5½oz each

Juice 1 lemon (optional)

Pre heat the oven to 180ºC/ 350ºF/Gas 4

1   Heat the olive oil in a saucepan or frying pan. Add the onion and garlic sauté for 3 – 4 minutes.

2   Add the chilli or Sambol Oelek, the cardamom, the cumin and the dill, give it a good stir and then add the tinned tomatoes and the tomato purée. Leave the sauce to cook gently over a low heat while you prepare the fish.

3   Wash and dry the fish and put it into a greased baking dish that is large enough to lay the fish in a single layer. Pour over the tomato sauce. Cover with foil and bake in the middle of the oven for 20 - 25 minutes depending on the thickness of the fish. The fish should be set and translucent.

Curried Fish Baked in Banana Chillies

*A smooth spicy coconut 'custard' with fish is used to fill large mild
chillies. If you are unable to obtain large chillies, use long sweet Ramiro
peppers or ordinary red or yellow bell peppers instead.*

SERVES 4

8 large banana chillies or 4 long
sweet Ramiro peppers

I red chilli finely sliced to garnish (optional)

Fish Filling:
1 tbsp red Thai curry paste
350g/12oz white fish
400ml/14fl oz coconut milk

8 large basil leaves
2 large free range eggs
2 tbsp Thai fish sauce
4 spring onions finely sliced
2 tbsp Japanese panko breadcrumbs

1   Pre heat the oven to 180°C/ 350°F/Gas 4

2   Combine the coconut milk, curry paste and eggs, the Thai fish
    sauce, spring onions and breadcrumbs and put to one side while
    the breadcrumbs soften and absorb some of the coconut milk.

3   Make a long slit in each of the chillies or peppers, put them onto a
    microwave dish and microwave on full power for 3 - 4 minutes.
    This will soften them a little and make them easier to de-seed.
    When the chillies or peppers are cool enough to handle open
    them up and remove the seeds. Put one or two basil leaves inside
    each pepper.

4   Cut the fish into small 1cm/½ in pieces and stir it into the coconut
    and egg mixture. Lay the chillies or peppers in a single layer in a
    large oven proof dish and spoon in the coconut and fish mixture.
    Cover with foil and bake for 20 minutes until the custard is set and
    the chillies or peppers are tender.

Fish Baked with Gremolata Crust

Gremolata is a very useful ingredient to have available so it is worthwhile keeping a supply of it in the freezer. You can use any type of white fish. Tilapia is ideal as it has a firm texture and it absorbs flavours really well.

SERVES 2

2 fillets of white fish weighing about 150g/5½oz each

70g/2½oz gremolata

1 tbsp finely chopped walnuts

3 tbsp toasted flaked oats

1 clove garlic crushed

1 tbsp finely grated parmesan

1 tbsp lemon juice

Pre heat the oven to 180°C/ 350°F/Gas 4

1   Mix together the gremolata, chopped walnuts, garlic, lemon juice, parmesan and toasted flaked oats.

2   Wash and dry the fish. Lay it onto a non stick baking tray or a sheet of oiled foil.

3   Scatter over the gremolata crumbs and bake for 20 minutes until the fish is set and translucent.

Fish Salad With Chive Vinaigrette

*This is one of those really simple 'naughty but nice' recipes that you
only eat once in a while. Skate or monk fish are the perfect fish to use
but any type of firm white fish will do. You need firm, waxy salad
potatoes for this dish and they need to be cooked and left to get cold
before using them.*

SERVES 4

600g/1lb 5oz firm white fish

Juice of a lemon

600g/1lb 5oz cooked waxy salad potatoes

50g/1¾oz rocket or baby spinach leaves

Ground black pepper to taste

3 tbsp white wine vinegar

30g/1oz butter

1 tbsp Thai fish sauce

4 tbsp finely chopped chives

Pre heat the oven to 200°C/ 400°F/Gas 5

1   Wash and dry the fish and lay it flat on a dish or baking tray.
    Season it with pepper and sprinkle over 1 or 2 tablespoons of
    lemon juice. Cover with foil and bake for 20 – 25 minutes until the
    flesh is firm and translucent. Take it out of the oven and leave it to
    cool.

2   Cut the fish into bite size pieces. Slice the potatoes into 5mm/¼ in
    rounds. Mix the potatoes, fish and rocket together and put it onto
    serving plates.

3   Melt the butter in a small saucepan and stir in the wine vinegar, 2
    tbsp lemon juice, the Thai fish sauce and the chives. Pour this over
    the fish potatoes and serve straight away.

Fish Pie with Rosti Potato Topping

You can use this fish pie mixture in a many different ways. You can use it to stuff peppers and courgettes and it also makes a good topping for a large family size omelette.

Use any type of fish and seafood depending on what you have available. This recipe uses leeks but courgettes and fennel work just as well. The basic rule is that you need about 150g/5½ oz fish per serving. As the pie mix freezes well it is worth making a large batch and freezing it in meal size portions.

SERVES 4

500g/1lb 2oz white fish skin and bones removed	2 tbsp dry vermouth or Noilly Prat
150g/5½oz prawns	1 tbsp Thai fish sauce
200g/7oz salmon skin and bones removed	425ml/15fl oz (¾pt) milk
200g/7oz leek white only finely sliced	For the topping
1 tsp dried dill	900g/2 lb potatoes peeled
Juice ½ lemon	1 tbsp capers dried and roughly chopped
55g/2oz butter	50g/1¾oz melted butter
1 tbsp flour	50g/1¾oz finely grated parmesan

You will need a 1½ Lt/2¾pt baking dish at least 5cm/2 in deep.

1. If the fish has been frozen wash and dry it carefully. Cut it into 1cm/½ in size pieces.

2. Put the leeks into a microwave bowl, cover and microwave for 5 minutes. Put them to one side while you make the sauce.

3. Pre heat the oven to 200ºC/ 400ºF/Gas 5

4. Melt the butter in a saucepan on a medium heat. When it is foaming add the flour and use a hand whisk to stir it while it cooks for a minute or two. Add the milk and stir with the whisk until the sauce thickens. Add the vermouth or Noilly Prat, the lemon juice,

dill and Thai fish sauce.

5   Turn down the heat to very low and leave the sauce to simmer while you prepare the potato topping.

6   Grate the potatoes and put them into a large bowl. Then stir in the cheese, capers and melted butter.

7   Grease the baking dish. Stir the cooked leeks into the sauce and then add the fish and prawns.

8   Turn off the heat and pour the fish and sauce into the baking dish. Scatter the potatoes on top and bake for 35 – 40 minutes.

Serve with a green salad, French beans or broccoli.

Fish Baked with Onion & Lemon Confit

You can prepare the onion confit used in this dish in advance and store it in the fridge for a day or two. It also freezes well so it is worth making more than you need and putting some in the freezer for emergency use. You can serve the baked fish with any type of green vegetable.

SERVES 4

350g/12oz white onion very
finely sliced
4 cloves of garlic finely chopped
50g/1¾oz unsalted butter or ghee
75ml/2½ fl oz dry white wine.
Finely grated zest of a lemon
Juice of a lemon
Parsley, chervil or dill to garnish.

3 bay leaves
150ml/5 fl oz (¼ pt) fish stock
4 fillets of white fish weighing about
150g/5½oz each, skin and bones removed
400g/14oz butter beans drained and rinsed

You will need a large flame proof casserole or baking dish to cook this as the fish needs to be cooked in a single layer. If you do not have any fish stock use vegetable stock and a tablespoon of Thai fish sauce.

1   Use a potato peeler to thinly peel 3 pieces of rind from the lemon. Cut this into fine, paper thin slices. Grate the rest of the lemon rind.

2   Melt the butter in a saucepan and add the onion, garlic, bay leaves and grated lemon rind. Sauté over a medium heat for 5 minutes, then add the white wine. Cover and leave to cook very slowly over a low heat for 40 minutes. Stir it occasionally to prevent the onions sticking.

3   Pre heat the oven to 220°C/ 450°F/Gas 6.

4   Wash and dry the fish.

5   Remove the bay leaves and add the butter beans and the fish stock to the onions. Bring them to the boil and turn off the heat.

6 Pour the onion and stock into the casserole, place the pieces of fish on top and sprinkle on the thin slices of lemon. Cover with a lid or foil and bake for 25 minutes.

To serve, put a piece of fish on each plate, stir the lemon juice into the onion and butter beans and put a spoonful onto the plate. Garnish with chopped dill, parsley or chervil.

Gremolata Prawns

The recipe for Gremolata is in the Herbs and Spices section. If the prawns are frozen thaw them out slowly and wash and dry them carefully. Serve the prawns with some noodles or a cucumber and potato salsa and a green salad. You will need large prawns with their shells still on and a wok or large frying pan to cook this.

SERVES 4

24 large unpeeled raw prawns that have been de-veined	50g/1¾oz ready made gremolata
	Juice ½ lemon
2 – 3 tbsp olive oil	Chopped flat leaf parsley or chervil to
2 cloves garlic crushed	garnish

1 Add the crushed garlic to the gremolata and put to one side.

2 Wash and dry the prawns.

3 Heat the olive oil in a wok or large frying pan. Add the prawns and cook them over a high heat for 4 to 5 minutes, stirring to prevent them sticking.

4 Take the prawns off the heat, stir in the gremolata, squeeze over the lemon juice and garnish with the parsley or chervil.

Tilapia Baked with Ginger, Soy & Sesame
You can use any type of white fish for this recipe.

SERVES 4

4 fillets of Tilapia each weighing
about 150g/5½oz

2 tbsp grated ginger

1 tbsp soy sauce

1 heaped tbsp toasted sesame
seeds

3 cloves garlic crushed

2 spring onions chopped

2 tsp sesame oil

1 tbsp olive oil

Juice of a lemon

Pre heat the oven to 200°C/ 400°F/Gas 5

1   Heat the oil in a small saucepan, add the garlic, ginger and spring
    onions and sauté over a medium heat for 2 – 3 minutes. Be careful
    not to let them brown.

2   Turn off the heat and mix in the soy sauce, sesame seeds, sesame
    oil and lemon juice. Put a quarter of the mixture into a small dish.

3   Wash and dry the fish and cut the fillets in half lengthways. If you
    are using tilapia you will have one thick piece and one thin piece.

4   Put a large piece of foil onto a baking sheet and lightly brush it
    with oil. Put the thick pieces of fish onto the foil, divide the sesame
    and ginger mixture between them and spread it out over the fillet.
    Put the thin pieces of fish on top and divide the rest of the sesame
    and ginger mixture between them.

5   Cover with foil, put it into the middle of the oven and bake for 25
    minutes.

Tamarind Prawns

This recipe uses fresh tomatoes but you can also use a can of chopped tomatoes. If you do not have any tamarind use the finely grated zest and juice of a lime instead. Instructions for making the tamarind pulp are in the Herbs and Spices section.

SERVES 4

1 medium onion thinly sliced
1 tbsp olive oil
1 tbsp grated ginger
2 cloves garlic crushed
4 tbsp tamarind pulp
Juice 1 lime
24 large prawns shelled and
de-veined

1 tbsp muscavado sugar
75ml/2½ fl oz water
1 tbsp Thai fish sauce
700g/1 lb 9oz tomatoes coarsely chopped
60g/2¼oz baby spinach leaves

1   Heat the oil and sauté the onion over a medium heat until it is soft.

2   Add the ginger and garlic and cook for 2 to 3 minutes. Be careful not to let the garlic burn.

3   Add the tamarind, sugar and water and bring to the boil, then stir in the tomatoes. Cover and simmer for 20 minutes until the mixture has thickened.

4   Add the prawns and cook, stirring occasionally, for 5 to 6 minutes. The prawns will change colour and become translucent

5   Stir in the baby spinach leaves and when these have wilted squeeze over the lime juice. Serve immediately.

Mussel & Prawn Curry

*Yellow Thai curry is made from chillies, turmeric, ginger and garlic. As
all of these are strongly anti-inflammatory, a yellow Thai curry makes a
healthy anti-inflammatory meal. You can buy Thai curry paste on line
and in Asian supermarkets. If you want to make your own, a recipe is
included in the Herbs and Spices section.*

SERVES 4

600ml/1 pt coconut milk

2 tbsp yellow curry paste or more to taste

1 tbsp Thai fish sauce

350g/12oz raw prawns, shelled and
de-veined

1 tbsp olive oil

200g/7oz mussel meat

12 baby onions or banana shallots peeled

250g/9oz cherry tomatoes

To garnish:

1 finely sliced red chilli

A handful of fresh coriander roughly
chopped

1   Bring the coconut milk gently to the boil. Add the curry paste and
    stir until the paste is dissolved. Bring to the boil, cover, reduce the
    heat and simmer for 5 minutes.

2   Taste the coconut sauce and if it is too spicy add a teaspoon of
    sugar. Add the shallots, bring the sauce back to the boil and
    simmer for 5 minutes.

3   Add the cherry tomatoes and the mussel meat, bring the curry
    sauce back to the boil, turn down the heat and leave it simmering
    while you cook the prawns.

4   Heat the olive oil in a wok and stir fry the prawns on a high heat
    for 3 to 4 minutes. The prawns are cooked when the flesh becomes
    translucent.

5   Add the curry sauce and the mussels to the prawns. Turn off the
    heat and garnish with the finely sliced chilli and the coriander.

Mussels with Coriander & Cumin

This recipe uses large green lip mussels in their shells. These are fresh water mussels that have a very different flavour to salt water mussels. You can usually buy them frozen in supermarkets. The mussels are already cooked. You can either grill the mussels or bake them in the oven.

SERVES 4

24 large green lip mussels in half shells

4 tbsp toasted oatmeal

50g/1¾oz coriander pesto

1 clove garlic crushed

½ tsp ground cumin

½ cayenne pepper

2 tbsp olive oil

Chopped coriander, parsley or chervil to garnish

Pre heat the oven to 200°C/ 400°F/Gas 5

1. Thaw the mussels slowly, then wash and dry them.

2. Mix the coriander pesto, crushed garlic, cayenne pepper and cumin with the olive oil and stir in the toasted oatmeal.

3. Line a baking sheet with non stick foil and arrange the mussels in a single layer open side up.

4. Divide the oatmeal and pesto mixture between the mussels and cook for 5 to 6 minutes until they are heated through.

Serve garnished with the chopped herbs.

Potato, Tomato & Mussel Bake

Use frozen mussel meat or fresh mussels in their shells. If you use fresh mussels you will need about 1Kg/2 lb 4oz of mussels and you will need to cook them and remove their shells first. This dish is best eaten hot, straight from the oven.

SERVES 4

450g/1lb mussel meat

450g/1lb potatoes

2 tbsp olive oil

2 cloves of garlic crushed

50g/1¾oz basil pesto

A hand full of basil leaves roughly torn

Crushed black pepper to taste

500g/1lb 2oz tomatoes skinned and thinly sliced

3 tbsp toasted oatmeal coating

Pre heat the oven to 180°C/ 350°F/Gas 4

1   Grease a shallow casserole or gratin dish.

2   Mix the olive oil with the crushed garlic.

3   Peel and slice the potatoes into 5mm/¼ in slices. Put them into a pan of boiling water, bring them to the boil and simmer them for 5 minutes. Drain the potatoes and arrange them in a single layer over the bottom of the casserole.

4   Arrange the mussels on top of the potatoes and drizzle the garlic and oil over them. Add the torn basil leaves.

5   Cover the mussels with the tomatoes and sprinkle over some crushed black pepper.

6   Mix the toasted oatmeal coating with the pesto and spoon this over the tomatoes.

7   Bake for 20 minutes until the tomatoes and potatoes are soft.

Prawns With Vegetable & Coconut Broth

This is a substantial main course. A platter of prawns, vegetables and noodles are served with a thick, spicy coconut broth. The recipe has a long list of ingredients and it looks complicated but it is actually simple to make and everything can be prepared in advance. You will need a large platter to serve this. You will find the recipe for nut butter in the Herbs and Spices section.

SERVES 4

2 tbsp ready made nut butter OR
40g/1½ oz raw nuts
4 shallots finely chopped
2 tbsp olive oil
Zest and juice of 1 lime
2 cloves garlic crushed
150g/5½oz thick rice noodles
1 tbsp olive oil
1cm/½ in cube shrimp paste OR
2 tbsp Thai fish sauce
1 tbsp mild curry powder
1 tbsp vegetable stock powder

400ml/14fl oz coconut milk
500ml/18fl oz raw or cooked prawns
2 baby gem lettuce OR 1 sweet Romaine lettuce finely shredded
150g/5½oz bean sprouts washed and drained
8 spring onions finely shredded
1 telegraph cucumber de-seed and cut into batons

1   Follow the instructions on the packet to cook the noodles. Drain and rinse them and stir in a tablespoon of olive oil to prevent them sticking together.

2   Arrange the shredded lettuce, cucumber, spring onions, bean sprouts and noodles in neat piles around the serving platter.

3   Mix the nut butter with the crushed garlic, lime zest and onions. If you are using nuts grind them in a blender.

4   To make the coconut broth, heat the olive oil in a wok or large saucepan and add the nuts, shallots and garlic. Sauté over a medium heat for 2 minutes. Add the shrimp paste or Thai fish

sauce, the curry powder, coconut milk and vegetable stock powder. Mix well and simmer for 10 minutes.

5   Add the prawns to the coconut broth, bring the broth back to the boil and simmer them for 4 to 5 minutes. If the prawns were raw they should become translucent and turn pink.

6   Take the prawns out and put them onto the serving platter in the middle of the vegetables.

7   Pour the coconut broth into a tureen or large bowl and serve it with the prawns and vegetables.

EGGS & LOW FAT DAIRY PRODUCTS

Eggs are mildly inflammatory, but they are also an excellent source of protein and essential fatty acids. In fact when it comes to valuable nutrients there is very little that eggs do not contain. However, in order to ensure that you have a healthy ratio of Omega-3 to Omega-6 make sure you buy free range eggs from hens that spend their life running around in a field. The nutritional content of a free range egg, especially its Omega-3 content, is totally different to an egg from a hen that is kept in a battery farm. You do not need to buy Omega-3 enriched eggs either. All this means is that the poor battery hen has been fed on fish meal. The eggs from the happy hens will have just as much Omega-3.

Eggs are bad for me, they contain a large amount of cholesterol? *Yes it is true, they do contain a large amount of cholesterol. A large boiled eggs weighs around 50 grams and it contains around 200mg of cholesterol. The same 50 gram portion of lean beef contains around 40mg. It's the old myth about saturated fats. Eggs contain a lot of healthy things as well as cholesterol. If they form part of a diet that is rich in antioxidants, vitamins, minerals and anti inflammatory foods they are fine.*

As long ago as the 17th Century the gout patient was told that milk was a good thing to drink. Now science has proved that it really is. Low fat diary products in the form of both milk and yoghurt are mildly inflammatory but despite this they are an essential part of a gout diet. But by yoghurt I mean natural unflavoured yoghurt that is not sweetened, not thickened and not pasteurised. It needs to be 'alive and kicking' with acidophilus, bifidus and other probiotics. Unless you have a major gastrointestinal imbalance you don't need to go out and buy 'probiotic' products, especially as the jury is still out on them. If the yoghurt is alive and not pasteurised and homogenised it will be brimming with the healthy bacteria your digestive tract needs.

However, remember that a surprisingly large number of people are allergic or have a level of intolerance to dairy products. If you are one of these, low fat diary will simply fuel the inflammation that already exists so avoid them like the plague. You could also try sheep or goat milk products which are often more easily tolerated.

CONTENTS

Egg Soubise

Soubise is a thick creamy sauce that is traditionally made with onions and cream. This recipe is quick and easy to prepare. It can be served with any type of vegetable or a simple salad. Without the boiled eggs the soubise will keep in the fridge for a couple of days. It can also be frozen. You can if you wish add some cooked mussels to the soubise just before you put it into the oven. This works particularly well if the soubise is made from leeks instead of onions. The large amount of onions used in this recipe makes this a good anti-inflammatory dish.

SERVES 4

750g/1lb 10oz white onions sliced
1 tbsp butter
3 tbsp milk
Finely grated zest and juice of ½ lemon
2 bay leaves
2 tbsp Japanese panko breadcrumbs

300ml/10 fl oz (½pt) fromage frais or Greek style natural unsweetened yoghurt
6 large free range eggs that have been hard boiled.
Crushed black pepper to taste

1   Heat the butter in a saucepan and gently sauté the onions over a medium heat for 5 minutes. Stir in the milk, the bay leaves and lemon zest, cover the saucepan, reduce the heat to low and simmer the onions for 30 minutes until they are soft. Leave them to cool slightly.

2   Pre heat the oven to 180°C/ 350°F/Gas 4

3   Peel the eggs and cut them in half. Put them cut side down either in individual dishes or in a single layer in a baking dish.

4   Remove the bay leaves and add the yoghurt, crushed black pepper and lemon juice to the onions. Purée them using a hand blender. Stir in the breadcrumbs and pour the purée over the eggs. Bake for 20 minutes.

Eggs in a Coconut Curry Sauce

A quick and easy way to serve eggs. For a healthy low carbohydrate option serve the curry with cauliflower 'rice'.

SERVES 4

8 large free range eggs

1 large white onion finely sliced

1 tbsp olive oil

1 small chilli finely chopped OR 2 tsp Sambol Oelek or chilli paste

2 cloves of garlic crushed

400ml/14fl oz can coconut milk

3 large tomatoes cut into quarters

2 tbsp finely grated ginger

1 tsp turmeric

2 tsp ground coriander

½ tsp ground green cardamom

3 tbsp fresh coriander chopped

1 large cauliflower, white only

1   Sauté the sliced onion in the olive oil for 5 minutes. Add the garlic, chilli, turmeric, cardamom and ground coriander. Cook for a minute or two and then add the coconut milk, grated ginger and tomatoes. Bring to the boil, reduce the heat and leave the sauce to simmer while you cook the eggs and cauliflower.

2   Boil the eggs for 12 minutes. Peel them, cut them in half and add them to the curry sauce.

3   Break the cauliflower into florets and cook it in boiling water for 3 to 4 minutes until it is just tender. Drain it and use a potato ricer or hand blender to mash it into a rough grainy texture.

4   Sprinkle the chopped coriander onto the egg curry just before serving with the cauliflower 'rice'.

Tofu with Scrambled Egg & Chilli

*This is one of those super quick meals that you can have ready in
minutes. You will need firm tofu or tempeh to make this.*

SERVES 4

2 tsp finely grated lemon zest

1 tbsp light soy sauce

1 tbsp rice vinegar

1 tbsp lemon juice

1 tsp sugar

1 clove garlic crushed

250g/9oz firm tofu

1 tbsp fine polenta for dusting

1 tbsp olive oil

1 red chilli finely sliced OR 1tsp Sambol
Oelek

1 red pepper finely diced

4 large free range eggs beaten

sliced red chilli or red pepper to garnish.

1 Combine the lemon zest, light soy sauce, rice vinegar, lemon juice
   and sugar in a bowl.

2 Cut the tofu into bite size pieces about 1cm/½in thick. If you have
   time, marinade it in the lemon and soy mixture for half an hour.
   Drain and dry it and lightly dust it with polenta.

3 Heat the oil in a wok or frying pan and cook the tofu over a high
   heat to seal it.

4 Remove the tofu from the pan and add the red pepper and chilli.
   Stir fry for 2 minutes, then add the crushed garlic, keeping
   everything moving so that the garlic does not go brown and burn.

5 Add the marinade mixture, stir and add the beaten eggs and the
   tofu.

6 Reduce the heat and cook very slowly until the eggs are just set.
   Garnish with finely sliced red chilli or red pepper before serving.

Vegetable Torte

This is somewhere between a pastry-less quiche and a terrine. You can make it with more or less any vegetables that you have available. The torte will keep for up to 2 days in the fridge but it will not freeze.

SERVES 6 - 8

250g/9oz courgette
250g/9oz cauliflower broken into
small florets
70g/2½oz fine French beans
1 medium white onion finely chopped
1 tbsp olive oil
2 cloves of garlic crushed

2 finely chopped preserved lemons
2 tbsp chopped basil
5 tbsp finely grated parmesan
200g/7oz feta
350g/12oz silken tofu
4 large free range eggs

Pre heat the oven to 160°C/325°F/Gas 3

1   Grease a 20cm/8 in cake tin and dust the inside with finely grated parmesan.

2   Sauté the onion and garlic in the olive oil over a medium heat for 5 minutes. Stir it occasionally, do not let it brown. Put them to one side.

3   Top and tail the French beans. Add them to a pan of boiling water and cook them for 3 – 4 minutes. Drain and refresh them in cold water.

4   Put the cauliflower into a large microwave bowl, add 3 tablespoons of water, cover and cook on full power for 3 minutes. Take the cauliflower out and put it to one side.

5   If the courgettes are large cut them in half lengthways and cut each half into 5mm/¼ in slices.

6   Put the sliced courgette and the mange tout into the microwave bowl, cover and cook for 3 minutes. Leave to cool.

7   Cut half of the feta into small 5mm/¼ in dice. Put the rest into a bowl with the tofu, eggs, chopped basil and the parmesan and blend everything together using a hand blender.

8   Stir in the onions, the vegetables, the chopped preserved lemons and diced feta.

9   Pour the mixture into the prepared cake tin, cover loosely with foil and bake in the centre of the oven for 45 minutes. Take the foil off and cook for another 15 minutes. Turn off the oven and leave the torte to cool before taking it out.

Omelettes

A classic omelette is quick and easy to make. You can fill it with a variety of different ingredients; sliced mushrooms that have been lightly sautéed, baby spinach leaves wilted with some chopped tomato and chilli, a handful of chives and mixed herbs and, strange as it may sound, a few spoonfuls of petite pois mixed with some wilted lettuce and lemon juice. The combinations are endless.

The technique is simple and success depends mainly on having a frying pan that is the right size for the number of eggs; if the pan is too big the omelette will be thin and tough, if it is too small it will be spongy and thick.

Eggs are inflammatory? Yes they are but only mildly and by adding just a tiny amount of chilli, cayenne pepper, garlic or turmeric you can balance out their inflammatory effect. Serve them with broccoli or a salad of baby spinach leaves and they provide a healthy nutritious anti-inflammatory meal.

Sardine Omelette

A strange combination but one that tastes really good and it is quick and easy to prepare. You can use any type of tinned oily fish to make this. Sardines work particularly well but make sure you use sardine fillets that have been canned in olive oil not sunflower oil.

SERVES 2

120g/4¼ oz sardine fillets in olive oil

5 large free range eggs

4 spring onions sliced OR half red onion finely chopped

Half finely chopped red chilli or ½ tsp chilli paste

1 large or 2 small tomatoes finely sliced.

1   Pour 1 tablespoon of the olive oil from the sardines into an omelette pan and drain the rest away. Break up the sardine fillets into large flakes.

2   Whisk the eggs until the whites and yolks are combined. Stir in the onions, the chopped chilli or chilli paste and the sardines.

3   Heat the grill on high.

4   Heat the oil in the omelette pan over a medium heat and pour in the eggs, tipping the eggs from side to side so that they are evenly spread.

5   Using a fork gently draw the edges of the egg towards the centre of the pan and let the liquid egg run to the edges. Keep doing this until the omelette is almost set but still moist on top.

6   Turn off the heat and put a layer of sliced tomatoes over the top of the omelette. Put it under the grill for 2 – 3 minutes until the tomatoes are heated through.

Serve immediately with some green vegetables or a green salad

Tortilla, Frittata & Kuku

A Kuku is a sort of solid unfolded omelette that contains vegetables and herbs. It is more like a Spanish tortilla or an Italian Frittata than a traditional omelette which should be lightly cooked and only just set in the centre. Kukus' originated in ancient Persia. It is hardly surprising that there is a similarity between the tortilla and the frittata as the kuku was brought to Spain by the Arabs and the spice traders brought it to Italy.

You can basically use more or less any vegetable to make kukus, tortillas and frittatas. Just make sure the ingredients are freshly cooked otherwise the finished dish will have a stale leftover taste. You can serve tortillas, frittatas and kukus hot or cold, as a main course, cut in slices for a picnic or cut into small squares as canapés. They make an excellent breakfast dish and they will keep for up to 2 days in a fridge.

Recipes for these types of egg dishes vary. Some add baking powder and some add flour, most are cooked slowly in a covered non stick frying pan. Whichever recipe you use and whichever way you choose to cook it, this type of egg dish provides a nutritious meal that is quick and easy to prepare.

Egg dishes of this type have a reputation of being a bit 'dried up'. Adding a small amount of cream, yoghurt or fromage frais helps prevent this. One thing you do need when making a tortilla, frittata or kuku is a high quality non stick frying pan, preferably one with a lid. If you can find one with a metal handle that you can put into the oven all the better as the easiest and fail safe way of cooking a tortilla or frittata is to start the process on the hob and then finish it in the oven.

Broccoli & Brie Frittata

You can make this with any type of broccoli and use either brie, Camembert or a soft goats log. You will need a 24cm/10 inch non stick frying pan that can go into the oven. Adding a small amount of yoghurt is optional but it does help to soften the tortilla and prevent it from becoming too hard.

SERVES 4

6 large free range eggs

3 tbsp natural unsweetened yoghurt (optional)

1 tbsp olive oil

400g/14oz tender stem or purple sprouting broccoli

175g/6oz brie or goats log

½ tsp garlic powder

¼ tsp ground turmeric

2 tbsp toasted pine nuts

Pre heat the oven to 180°C/ 350°F/Gas 4

1 Cook the broccoli for 3 minutes. Drain and put to one side to cool a little.

2 Cut the cheese into 1cm/½ in pieces.

3 Whisk the eggs and yoghurt in a large bowl with the turmeric and garlic powder. Season to taste with salt and pepper. Mix the broccoli, cheese and pine nuts into the eggs.

4 Heat the frying pan with 1 tsp olive oil over a medium heat and add the eggs, broccoli and cheese. Cook for 5 minutes then cover it and put the pan into the oven. Cook for 20 minutes.

5 Pre heat the grill to high. Take the frying pan out of the oven, remove the lid and pop it under the grill until the top of the tortilla is set. Serve at once.

Cauliflower, Tomato & Anchovy Frittata

This is frittata makes a substantial family meal. You can eat it hot, cold or at room temperature.

SERVES 4

6 large free range eggs

3 tbsp natural unsweetened yoghurt (optional)

2 cloves garlic crushed

1 tsp chilli paste, chilli flakes or Sambol Oelek

1 medium cauliflower broken into small florets

150g/5½oz cherry tomatoes cut in half

4 spring onions sliced

50g/1¾oz tin anchovy fillets

2 – 3 tbsp capers drained and rinsed

10 salted black olives, stones removed

You will need a 24cm/10 in non stick frying pan or chefs pan with a lid to make this. Pre heat the oven to 180ºC/ 350ºF/Gas 4

1. Cook the cauliflower for 3 - 4 minutes. Drain and put to one side to cool a little.

2. Whisk the eggs in a large bowl with the Sambol Oelek, crushed garlic and yoghurt. Stir in the cauliflower, tomatoes, sliced spring onions, black olives and capers.

3. Pour 1 tbsp of the olive oil from the anchovies into the frying pan and heat it over a medium heat. Pour in the egg and cauliflower mixture and cook for 5 minutes then cover it and put the pan into the oven. Cook for 20 minutes.

4. Pre heat the grill to high. Take the frying pan out of the oven, remove the lid and arrange the anchovy fillets on top. Pop it under the grill and cook for 3 – 4 minutes until the top of the tortilla is set and the anchovies have cooked through.

Variations To Basic Tortilla & Frittata Mix

To 6 eggs and 3 tbsp natural unsweetened yoghurt add:

Potato and Za-atar

400g cooked sliced salad potatoes, 4 finely sliced spring onions, 1 crushed clove of garlic and 1 tsp za-atar.

After the tortilla is cooked put 100g crumbled feta and another teaspoon of za-atar on top of the tortilla before putting it under a hot grill for a couple of minutes.

Pumpkin, Spinach and Walnut

750g/1lb 10oz pumpkin cut into 2cm/1 in chunks and baked until it is just tender, 200g/7 ox cooked spinach, 3 tbsp chopped walnuts or pecan nuts.

Aubergine Kuku

This is traditionally made with aubergines that are skinned after they are cooked. However, leaving the skin on improves the texture as well as the colour of this dish.

SERVES 4

4 Aubergines weighing about ¾ Kg coarsely chopped	2 heaped tbsp fine polenta OR flour
2 large white onions coarsely chopped	Crushed black pepper to taste
2 tbsp olive oil or clarified butter	2 - 3 tbsp lemon juice
4 large eggs	

1 Cook the onions slowly in the butter or oil fro 10 minutes. Do not let them turn brown.

2 Add the aubergines and 1 or 2 tablespoons of water, cover with a lid and simmer slowly until the aubergines are soft. Mash them lightly and leave to cool a little.

3 Pre heat the oven to 200°C/ 400°F/Gas 5

4 Whisk the eggs and mix them with the aubergine, onion, pepper, lemon juice and the flour or polenta.

5 Grease a rectangular dish about 20cm x 25cm/8" x 10", pour in the aubergine and egg mixture and smooth over the top. Bake for 30 minutes. The kuku should be just set.

Cut the kuku into squares and serve, hot or at room temperature.

Terrines

Terrines may sound a bit grand but they are much easier to make than you think. They can be served hot or cold, as a starter or as a main course. They will keep for a couple of days in the fridge but they do not freeze.

Most of the recipes you see for terrines use cream but you can make a healthier option with low fat cheese such as quark and ricotta, natural unsweetened yoghurt and silken tofu.

Because they are 'delicate' terrines are traditionally cooked in a bain-marie; a tin or baking dish of hot water that you stand the terrine in while it is being cooked. However, by adding a small amount of fine polenta or panko (Japanese) breadcrumbs you can make the terrine robust enough to cook it in an ordinary oven without the bain-marie.

However, the easiest and most convenient way of cooking a terrine is in a microwave. Cooking times very depending on the power of the microwave. As a guide, most of the terrines in the recipes below will take about 30 minutes if the microwave is set on medium or 50% power. The terrine is cooked when it is firm to touch in the centre. Leave the terrine to stand for at least 10 minutes before turning it out.

Cheese & Vegetable Terrine

A simple terrine that uses basic ingredients. Use any type of hard cheese to make this, but finely grated parmesan gives the best flavour. Butternut squash or sweet potato can be used instead of the carrot. You will find the recipe for the nut butter in the Herbs and Spices section.

You will need a 1.4 Lt/2½ pt silicon loaf tin or a glass loaf tin lined with non stick parchment to make this.

SERVES 4 – 6

350g/12oz carrots peeled	3 tbsp parsley finely chopped
350g/12oz courgettes grated	For the nut sauce:
350g/12 oz leeks finely sliced	3 tbsp almond, walnut, pecan nut or cashew
1 clove garlic crushed	nut butter.
1 tsp ground turmeric	150ml/¼ pt natural unsweetened yoghurt
3 large free range eggs beaten	1 tsp cornflour
350g/12oz silken tofu	2 tbsp Noilly Prat or dry vermouth
3 tbsp finely grated parmesan	(optional)
50g/1¾oz polenta OR panko (Japanese) breadcrumbs	Salt and pepper to taste

1   Coarsely grated the carrot and put it with the courgettes, leek and garlic into a microwave bowl. Cover and cook on high power for 3 minutes. Stir the vegetables and cook them for another 2 minutes. Put them to one side and leave them to cool slightly.

2   Put the silken tofu, turmeric and eggs into a large bowl and blend with a hand blender until you have s smooth mixture. Add the breadcrumbs or polenta, the parsley and cheese and season to taste with salt and pepper. Stir in the carrot, courgettes and leek and mix well.

3   Turn the mixture into the prepared loaf tin and level the surface. Cover with cling film and leave it to stand for 15 minutes before putting it in the microwave.

4   Cook on 50 % power for 30 minutes. The terrine is cooked when it is firm to the touch in the centre. Leave the terrine to stand for at least 10 minutes before turning it out.

5   To make the nut sauce, put the yoghurt into a microwave bowl and whisk in the cornflour and dry vermouth. Stir in the nut butter and microwave on full power for 3 – 4 minutes.

Crab Terrine

You can use fresh or frozen crab to make this and use courgettes, leeks or fennel as the base. If you want to turn this into a salmon terrine use 200g/7oz of white fish and 300g/10½ oz cooked salmon. You will need a 1.4 Lt/2½ pt silicon loaf tin or a glass loaf tin lined with non stick parchment or foil to make this.

SERVES 4 – 6

300g/10½ oz white fish

Brown and white meat from a

500g/1lb 2oz brown crab

3 large free range eggs

½ tsp cayenne pepper

300g/10½oz coarsely grated courgette

175ml/6fl oz natural unsweetened yoghurt

Zest ½ lemon finely grated

Juice 1 lemon

1 tbsp fresh dill OR 1 tsp dried dill

2 tbsp spring onion green OR 2 tbsp chopped chives

1 tbsp Thai fish sauce

50g/1¾oz fine polenta

1   Wash and dry the fish and chop it up into chunks. Put it into a blender or food processor with the eggs, polenta, cayenne pepper and yoghurt. Blitz until blended.

2   Turn the mixture into a large mixing bowl. Stir in the dried dill, the grated lemon zest and the lemon juice. Now stir in the grated courgette, the spring onion and the Thai fish sauce and then the brown and white crab meat.

3   Put the mixture into the prepared tin, level the surface, cover with cling film and leave it to stand for at least 15 minutes before putting it into the microwave.

4   Cook on 50% power for 30 minutes. The terrine is cooked when it is firm to the touch in the centre. Leave the terrine to cool completely before turning it out.

Prawn Terrine

You can use fresh or frozen prawns to make this. This recipe uses courgettes but you could also use leeks or fennel. The terrine is best eaten cold. It will keep for up to 2 days in the fridge.

You will need a 1.4 Lt/2½ pt silicon loaf tin or an glass loaf tin lined with non stick parchment to make this.

SERVES 4 – 6

400g/14 oz courgettes coarsely grated
250g/9oz shelled prawns
250g/9 oz tub of quark or ricotta
3 large free range eggs
1 tbsp fresh dill OR 1 tsp dried dill
Finely grated zest of half a lemon

1 tbsp Thai fish sauce
3 – 4 spring onions finely sliced
50g/1¾oz polenta OR panko (Japanese) breadcrumbs

1   Mix the eggs, dried dill, lemon zest, quark or ricotta and Thai fish sauce together using a hand blender.

2   Stir in the grated courgettes and spring onions and mix well. Add the prawns and the breadcrumbs or polenta.

3   Put the mixture into the prepared tin, level the surface, cover with cling film and leave it to stand for at least 15 minutes before putting it in the microwave.

4   Cook on 50% power for 30 minutes.

5   The terrine is cooked when it is firm to the touch in the centre. Leave the terrine to cool completely before turning it out.

Roulades

*A roulade is basically a thin soufflé that is rolled up around a filling.
They look impressive and they are surprisingly easy to make. Like
terrines roulades do not freeze well but most can be stored in the fridge
for up to two days.*

Brazil Nut Roulade.

*Just about all nuts are anti-inflammatory and Brazil nuts come top of
the list. This is a really simple recipe that you can use as a base for
many different types of roulade. A similar roulade made with hazelnuts
and chocolate is included in the section on desserts.*

*This recipe uses cannellini beans, soft cheese and roasted red peppers
as the filling but you can fill the roulade with any combination of soft
cheese and vegetable. The roulade will keep for up to 2 days in the
fridge.*

SERVES 6 – 8

175g/6oz finely ground Brazil nuts
30g/1oz flaked oats
4 large free range eggs
½ crushed clove garlic (optional)

400g/14oz can cannellini beans drained
and rinsed
100g/3½oz Ricotta, Quark or cream goats
cheese
3 roasted red peppers cut into strips

Filling:
2 - 3 tbsp finely sliced chives

Pre heat the oven to 200°C/ 400°F/Gas 5 and line a 32cm (13in) x
23cm (9in) Swiss roll tin with non stick baking parchment or non stick
foil.

1   Cut the red peppers in quarters and roast them for 30 minutes
    until their skin is beginning to blister and look charred. Put them
    into a dish, cover them with cling film and leave them to cool a
    little. When they are cool enough to handle peel the skins off of

the peppers and cut them into strips. Reserve any oil and juices that come out of the roasted peppers.

2   Put the Brazil nuts, flaked oats and, if you using it, the garlic into a food processor and process until the nuts are ground to a fine powder.

3   Separate the eggs and put the egg whites into a large, dry bowl. Whisk the egg whites until they form soft peaks. Add the egg yolks and quickly whisk them in. Don't over whisk or the mixture will lose its volume. Carefully fold in the ground nuts.

4   Pour the mixture onto the prepared Swiss roll tin and spread it out evenly. Bake in the middle of the oven for 8 – 10 minutes. It should be just firm to the touch and springy when cooked. Take it out of the oven and cover it with a sheet of baking parchment and a clean tea towel. Leave it to cool.

5   To make the filling, drain and rinse the cannellini beans and put them into a bowl with the soft cheese. Use a hand blender to mix them together into a smooth purée.

6   To assemble the roulade. Take off the tea towel, put a large board on top and turn the roulade over. Remove the baking parchment. Using a sharp knife, trim off the edges. You need to do this as it makes it easier to roll the roulade up.

7   Spread the bean and cheese mixture evenly over the roulade and arrange the slices of roasted pepper on top. Drizzle over the reserved pepper juices and sprinkle over the sliced chives.

Pick up the baking parchment along a long side of the roulade and gently roll the roulade over using the baking parchment to move it forward. Roll the roulade up in the baking parchment and put it into the fridge until you are ready to serve it.

Salmon & Spinach Roulade

*A simple roulade, that is made from leaf spinach that has been puréed.
It is worth keeping a few bags of ready prepared spinach purée in the
freezer to speed up the process of making this. You can use fresh or
frozen spinach.*

*You can fill the roulade with more or less anything. Cottage cheese,
oven dried tomatoes and black olives work well. This roulade is filled
with salmon pâté and prawns. The roulade will keep for up to 2 days in
the fridge.*

SERVES 6 – 8

200g/7oz cooked spinach	Filling
30g/1oz butter at room temperature	200g/7 oz silken tofu or soft low fat cheese
4 large free range eggs	like Quark or Ricotta
3 tbsp finely grated parmesan plus	1 – 2 tsp dried dill
1 tbsp for dusting	3 spring onions finely sliced
½ tsp grated nutmeg	300g/10½oz cooked salmon
Finely grated zest of half a lemon	100g/3½oz cooked prawns

Pre heat the oven to 190°C/ 400°F/Gas 5. and line a 32cm (13in) x
23cm (9in) Swiss roll tin with non stick baking parchment or non stick
foil.

1   Cook the spinach and squeeze out as much water as possible. The
best way of doing this is by using a sieve and/or your hands. Leave
it to cool.

2   To make the filling, put the salmon, cheese or tofu and dill into a
bowl and use a hand blender to mix it into a thick paste. Stir in the
spring onions. Cover and put it to one side.

3   Separate the eggs and put the whites into a large dry bowl.

4   Put the spinach into a blender or food processor and blend it until
you have a smooth purée. Now add the butter, grated nutmeg,

grated parmesan, lemon zest if using it and the egg yolks and blend until you have a smooth creamy looking purée. Put this into a large bowl.

5   Whisk the egg whites until they form soft peaks. Add a third of the whisked eggs to the spinach purée and mix them in using a metal spoon. Add the rest of the egg whites and gently fold them in. Pour the mixture into the lined Swiss roll tin and bake for 12 - 15 minutes. The top should feel springy when you touch it.

6   Scatter over the remaining tablespoon of grated parmesan and cover the roulade with a sheet of baking parchment and a clean tea towel. Leave it to cool.

7   To assemble the roulade. Take off the tea towel, put a large board on top and turn the roulade over. Remove the baking parchment from the underneath of the roulade. Using a sharp knife trim off the edges. You need to do this as it makes it easier to roll the roulade up.

8   Spread the salmon pâté over the roulade and scatter the prawns over it.

9   Pick up the baking parchment underneath the roulade along one of the long sides and gently roll the roulade over using the baking parchment to move it forward. Roll the roulade up and arrange it with the end underneath. Wrap it in the baking parchment and put it into the fridge until you are ready to serve it.

Carrot Roulade With Hummus

You can make this with carrot, butternut squash, pumpkin or sweet potato. It takes a bit longer to make than the spinach and Brazil nut roulade but it is worth the effort. Like the other roulades this will keep for up to 2 days in the fridge. You will find the recipe for black olive Tapenade in the Herbs and Spices section.

SERVES 6 – 8

280g/10oz grated carrot	½ -1 clove crushed garlic
50g/1¾oz butter	3 tbsp Tahini paste
50g/1¾oz plain flour	2 tbsp natural unsweetened yoghurt
4 free range eggs	2 tbsp lemon juice
300ml/10 fl oz (½pt) milk	Half packet washed ready to eat rocket
1 tbsp finely grated parmesan	
Filling:	
2 tbsp black olive tapenade	
400g can of chick peas that have been drained and rinsed.	

Pre heat the oven to 190ºC/ 400ºF/Gas 5 and line a 32cm (13in) x 23cm (9in) Swiss roll tin with non stick baking parchment or non stick foil.

1. Separate the eggs. Put the whites into a large dry bowl and the yolks into a small basin or cup.

2. Melt the butter in a saucepan over a medium heat and stir in the flour. Cook the flour and butter for 2 – 3 minutes over a low heat. Using a whisk stir in the milk and continue stirring until the sauce thickens. Turn off the heat and leave the sauce to cool slightly before mixing in the egg yolks.

3. Put the grated carrots into a large bowl and stir in the sauce.

4. Whisk the egg whites until they form soft peaks. Add a third of the

whisked egg white to the carrots and fold it in using a metal spoon. Now add this to the rest of the egg whites and gently fold it in. Pour the mixture into the lined Swiss roll tin and bake for 15 to 20 minutes. When it is cooked the top should be lightly browned and feel springy when you touch it.

5. Scatter over one tablespoon of grated parmesan and cover it with a sheet of baking parchment and a clean tea towel. Leave it to cool.

6. To make the filling, drain and rinse the chickpeas and put them with the garlic, Tahini, lemon juice and yoghurt into a bowl and whiz it with a hand blender until it has a smooth, creamy consistency.

7. To assemble the roulade. Take off the tea towel, put a large board on top and turn the roulade over. Remove the baking parchment from the underneath of the roulade.. Using a sharp knife trim off the edges. You need to do this as it makes it easier to roll the roulade up.

8. Spread the black olive tapenade over the roulade. On top of this spread the chick pea purée and then spread a layer of rocket on top.

9. Pick up the baking parchment underneath the roulade along one of the long sides and gently roll the roulade over using the baking parchment to move it forward. Roll the roulade up and arrange it with the end underneath. Wrap it in the baking parchment and put it into the fridge until you are ready to serve it.

GRAINS & RICE

All grains and cereals are inflammatory. Some are mildly inflammatory, some are moderately inflammatory and some are highly inflammatory. As a general rule the more refined the grain is the more inflammatory it becomes. However, this does not mean that you have to exclude grains and cereals form your diet. By combining them with ingredients that are anti-inflammatory you can create a balanced anti-inflammatory meal.

For anyone who is gluten intolerant quinoa, millet, rice, buckwheat and most oatmeal are much better to eat than bulgar wheat, spelt, barley and couscous as all of these contain gluten.

The recipes in this section use different types of grains but you can use more or less use any grain or cereal to make them. Some grains are easier to cook than others. Surprisingly all grains, including rice, can be frozen once they are cooked so it is worth keeping a supply of the grains that take a long time to cook in the freezer.

CONTENTS

Cooking Quinoa

Quinoa is not the easiest of grains to cook as it needs long, very slow cooking. The best way to cook it is by using the absorption method. One part quinoa needs just slightly under two parts of water. The easiest way to do this is to use a small 5fl oz/150 ml dish like a ramekin dish. This holds about 100g/3½ oz of quinoa. Even if the packet says the quinoa is already washed, wash and drain it again.

You can cook quinoa on the hob or in the microwave.

To cook it on the hob, put the quinoa into a saucepan, bring it to the boil, cover with a tight fitting lid and reduce to a very low heat. Leave it to cook for 25 – 30 minutes. When it has finished cooking leave it to stand for at least a quarter of an hour before taking off the lid.

To cook it in the microwave, put the quinoa into a microwave bowl with the water. Cover it loosely and microwave on full power for 10 minutes. Give it a stir, put the cover back on and leave it to stand for 10 minutes. Then microwave it again on full power for 4 minutes and leave it to stand for 3 – 4 minutes before serving.

Troublesome it may be to cook, but quinoa is packed full of protein and it has a low glycemic index. Of all of the grains it is probably the healthiest one to eat.

To freeze quinoa all you need to do is open freeze it on a large tray lined with cling film or non stick foil and when it is frozen put it into a box or a bag so that you can use it as and when needed. It thaws out very quickly once it is taken out of the freezer.

Cooking Millet
Like most grains the best way to cook millet is by using the absorption method. Like quinoa one part millet needs about two parts of water. The easiest way to do this is to use a small 5fl oz/150 ml ramekin dish. This holds about 100g/3½ oz of millet.

To cook it on the hob, put the millet into a saucepan, bring it to the boil, cover with a tight fitting lid and reduce to a very low heat. Leave it to cook for 35 – 40 minutes. When it has finished cooking add a tablespoon of boiling water, put the lid back on and leave it to stand for a quarter of an hour before taking off the lid.

Cooking Whole Buckwheat
Unlike millet and quinoa whole buckwheat is best covered with cold water, brought to the boil and then simmered very gently for between 20 to 25 minutes. Drain before serving.

Cooking Pearl Barley & Pearl Spelt
As with buckwheat these are best covered with cold water, brought to the boil and then simmered slowly. Make sure you wash the spelt or barley well before cooking it as it tends to be quite dusty. Pearl spelt needs to simmer for about 20 minutes but pearl barley will need to simmer for 50 minutes before it is cooked.

Cooking Couscous.
Couscous is made from wheat and sometimes barley. It comes in fine, medium and giant forms. Because it it pre-processed couscous is by far the easiest 'grain' to prepare. All you need to do is add 1 part couscous to 2 parts boiling water, give it a stir and then leave it to stand for 5 – 10 minutes. Medium couscous needs to be gently simmered for 5 minutes before being left to stand. Giant couscous needs to be simmered for 10 minutes.

Cooking Bulgar Wheat

Bulgar wheat is a whole cracked part processed wheat that like couscous comes in fine, medium and course varieties. It is cooked in exactly the same way as couscous.

For fine bulgar wheat add 1 part couscous to 2 parts boiling water, give it a stir and then leave it to stand for 5 – 10 minutes. Medium bulgar wheat needs to be gently simmered for 5 minutes before being left to stand. Course bulgar wheat needs to be simmered for 10 minutes.

Toasting Oatmeal

Having a supply of oatmeal that is already toasted is well worthwhile as it is a useful store cupboard ingredient. It is a good alternative to breadcrumbs for making toppings for gratins and it works really well when mixed with pesto as a topping. It can also be used in biscuits and deserts.

You can either grill the oatmeal or toast it in a dry pan on the hob.

To grill the oatmeal pre heat the grill on high and put the oatmeal in a thin layer on a tray. Grill under a high heat for 3 to 4 minutes, stirring it and turning it over every minute. Keep you eye on it as it burns very easily. When it is ready it should be a light golden brown.

To toast the oatmeal on the hob pre heat a pan over a medium heat and when it is hot put in the oatmeal. Keep stirring it around. It should take about 5 minutes to turn golden brown.

Once it has cooled down you will need to store the oatmeal in an airtight container.

Toasted Oatmeal Coating

This is a useful mixture of oatmeal, spices and seeds that can be used as a crunchy topping for bakes an gratins and as a coating for burgers.

SERVES 4

200g/7oz flaked oatmeal

3 tbsp olive oil

3 tbsp water

A handful of sunflower seeds

½ tsp ground turmeric

1 tsp garlic granules

1 tbsp dried oregano

1 tsp chilli flakes

Pre heat the oven to 160°C/ 325°F/Gas 3

Grease a 20cm/8 in square baking tin and line the base with baking parchment or non stick foil.

1. Mix the flaked oats and sunflower seeds with the turmeric, garlic granules, chilli flakes and oregano.

2. Put the water and olive oil into a saucepan and bring it to the boil.

3. Add the oil and water for the flaked oats. Mix well and press the mixture into the prepared tin. Bake for 30 minutes until the oats are golden brown.

4. Leave the oats to cool completely, then use a rolling pin to break the oats down into large crumbs.

5. Store in an airtight tin or freeze.

Kedgeree

Kedgeree is traditionally made from basmati rice and smoked haddock.
This recipe is made from buckwheat and smoked mackerel. It will taste
just as good if it is made with salmon, trout or smoked haddock and
instead of the buckwheat pearl spelt, rice, barley or quinoa. The nutty
taste of buckwheat works really well with the smoked mackerel.

SERVES 4

200g/7oz buckwheat

1 tsp turmeric

3 bay leaves

200g/7oz hot smoked mackerel

4 hard boiled eggs, peeled and cut into quarters

1 large white onion finely sliced

1 large stick of celery chopped

Juice of a lemon

2 tbsp olive oil

1 tsp ground cardamom

2 tbsp chopped dill

1 tbsp chopped parsley

100g/3½oz frozen peas

200g/7oz mange tout cut in half lengthways

You will need a large frying pan or a chefs pan with a lid to make this.

1. Put the buckwheat into a saucepan, add the turmeric and bay leaves, cover it with plenty of water and bring it to the boil. When the buckwheat is boiling reduce the heat, cover it and simmer it for 20 minutes. Drain, remove the bay leaves and put the buckwheat to one side.

2. Take the skin off of the smoked mackerel and break up the fillets into bite size pieces.

3. Heat the oil in a frying pan and sauté the onion and celery on a medium heat for 5 minutes until they are tender.

4. Add the ground cardamom and stir in the cooked buckwheat. Add 2 tbsp water and lay the pieces of mackerel on top. Put the lid on a leave the buckwheat and fish to heat through over a low heat for a

few minutes while you cook the peas and mange tout.

5. Put the peas into a microwave bowl with 2 tbsp water, cover and microwave on full power for 4 minutes. Add the mange tout, replace the cover and cook for another minute.

6. Strain the peas and mange tout and stir them into the mackerel and buckwheat. Turn off the heat, arrange the hard boiled eggs on top and scatter over the chopped dill and parsley.

Buckwheat Porcini & Chestnuts

*You can use buckwheat, pearl spelt, pearl barley or quinoa to make this.
You will need a large frying pan or a chefs pan with a lid.*

SERVES 4

200g/7oz buckwheat

200g/7oz chestnut mushrooms

200g/7oz cooked whole chestnuts

10g/¼ oz Porcini mushrooms

100ml/3½ fl oz water

1 tsp vegetable stock powder

3 cloves garlic finely shredded

1 large white onion finely sliced

½ tsp cayenne pepper

2 tbsp olive oil

200g/7oz baby spinach washed and
drained

3 tbsp finely grated parmesan

1   Put the Porcini mushrooms into a small saucepan with the
    vegetable stock powder and cayenne pepper. Cover them with
    100ml/3½ fl oz of water and bring them to the boil. Cover them,
    turn off the heat and leave them to soak while you cook the
    buckwheat.

2   Put the buckwheat into a saucepan, cover it with plenty of water
    and bring it to the boil. When it is boiling reduce the heat, cover it
    and simmer it for 15 minutes. Drain it and put it to one side.

3   Bring the Porcini mushrooms to the boil and leave them simmering
    over a low heat.

4   If the mushrooms are large slice them or cut them into halves or
    quarters. Heat the oil in a large frying pan, add the mushrooms
    and cook them for 5 minutes, stirring them once or twice.

5   Add the sliced onion and garlic to the mushrooms and cook over a
    medium heat for 5 minutes.

6   Add the Porcini mushrooms, the stock they were cooked in and the
    chestnuts. Bring everything to the boil, cover, reduce the heat and

simmer for 5 minutes.

7   Now add the buckwheat. Bring everything back to the boil and cook over a medium heat, stirring occasionally until most of the stock is absorbed.

8   Just before serving add half of the grated parmesan and the baby spinach and stir until the spinach is just wilted.

Serve the remaining parmesan in a separate bowl.

Mussel & Spelt Risotto

Use either pearl spelt, pearl barley, quinoa or risotto rice. You will need to adjust the cooking time accordingly. The basic risotto can be prepared in advance, kept in the fridge and finished when you are ready to eat it. You can substitute vegetable stock and a tablespoon of Thai fish sauce if you do not have any fish stock.

SERVES 4

200g/7oz pearl spelt

20g/½oz butter

200g/7oz white fish fillet with skin and bones removed

200g/7oz mussel meat

1Lt/1¾ pt/35 fl oz fish stock

2 tbsp finely chopped fresh dill or 2 tsp dried dill

1 tbsp finely grated lemon zest

8 spring onions finely sliced

2 tbsp dry vermouth or Noilly Prat

3 tbsp finely grated parmesan

2 tbsp thick fromage frais or natural Greek style yoghurt

Fresh dill, parsley or chervil to garnish

1 Wash and drain the spelt and put it into a pan with ¾ of the fish stock. Bring it to the boil, reduce the heat to low, cover and simmer for 15 minutes. Turn off the heat and put it to one side until you are ready to finish the dish.

2 Heat the remaining stock with the dill and lemon zest. Add the fish, turn down the heat to low, cover and simmer the fish for 4 – 5 minutes until it is opaque.

3 Take the fish out and put it to one side. Reserve the liquid the fish was cooked in.

4 To finish the risotto, Flake the fish and remove any bones.

5 Strain the stock the fish was cooked in and add it to the spelt, bring it to the boil and stir over a moderate heat until most of the stock is absorbed.

6   Stir in the butter and then add the dry vermouth, parmesan and yoghurt.

7   Season to taste with salt and pepper and gently stir in the fish, the mussels and the spring onions. Cook gently over a medium heat until the fish and mussels are heated through.

Serve garnished with the chopped fresh herbs.

Pumpkin Kibbeh

Kibbeh is a staple food in many Middle Eastern countries. It is usually made with meat and fine bulgar wheat that is shaped into rissoles and then fried in hot oil. This recipe uses pumpkin or butternut squash and, instead of being fried, the kibbeh is baked in the oven. If you are avoiding wheat products substitute quinoa for the bulgar wheat. The sumac used is this recipe has a sharp slightly acid taste. If you do not have any, use a tablespoon of tamarind pulp or an extra tablespoon of lemon juice instead.

You can serve Kibbeh hot, cold from the fridge or at room temperature. It freezes well and will keep in the fridge for up to 2 days.

SERVES 4 – 6

500g/1lb 2oz pumpkin or butternut squash peeled and cut into 2cm/1in pieces

100g/3½oz fine bulgar wheat

200ml/7 fl oz water

50g/1¾oz fine oatmeal

1 medium white onion grated

1 tsp ground cumin

1 tsp ground coriander

Crushed black pepper to taste

1 tbsp olive oil

100g/3½oz ready to eat apricots coarsely chopped

1 tsp sumac

Juice of a lemon

500g/1lb 2oz frozen spinach cooked and well drained

120g/4¼ oz feta or ricotta

1 preserved lemon finely chopped (optional)

For the filling:

2 shallots finely chopped

2 cloves of garlic crushed

1   Grease a 20cm/8 in square baking tin and line the base with baking parchment or non stick foil.

2   Put the bulgar wheat, cumin and coriander into a small saucepan, add 200ml/7 fl oz of water, bring it to the boil, cover and leave to cool.

3   Put the pumpkin into a microwave bowl, cover and cook on full power for 10 minutes. The pumpkin should be soft when tested with a sharp knife. Use a hand blender to mash the pumpkin into a smooth purée.

4   Add the finely grated onion, bulgar wheat and oatmeal to the puréed pumpkin, mix well and leave it to cool.

5   Cook the frozen spinach and drain it really well.

6   Sauté the chopped shallots and crushed garlic over a medium heat for 5 minutes. Stir in the cooked spinach, chopped apricots, the sumac and the lemon juice. Leave to cool.

Pre heat the oven to 180°C/ 350°F/Gas 4

7   Put half of the pumpkin mixture into the prepared tin and spread it over the base.

8   Cut the feta into 5mm/¼ in dice and mix it into the spinach mixture. Spread this evenly over the pumpkin and put the rest of the pumpkin mixture on top. Bake for 30 minutes in the middle of the oven.

Leave the Kibbeh to stand for 10 minutes before serving.

Oven Baked Beetroot Risotto

If lurid pink food is not to your liking then you may need to pass on this one. Despite its colour the recipe does taste really good and it is very easy to make.

Most recipes for risotto insist that the risotto must be stirred constantly while it is cooking, that the stock needs to be kept simmering and added slowly. This makes cooking a risotto somewhat tedious and as a consequence it puts people off making them. Well, we cook rice puddings in the oven so why not risotto?

The following recipe can be made either in the oven or on the hob. If you are making it in the conventional way allow about 20 minutes cooking time. If you are cooking it in the oven you will need to allow about 35 - 40 minutes.

SERVES 4

450g/1 lb cooked beetroot	½ tsp cayenne pepper
1 large white onion finely chopped	90g/3 ½oz finely grated parmesan or
30g/1 oz butter	pecorino
400g Arborio or other risotto rice	1 tbsp finely chopped parsley or chervil
3 cloves of garlic crushed	150g/5 oz firm goats cheese or crumbled
1.2Lt/2¼ pt vegetable stock	feta
Zest of half a lemon	
Juice of 1 lemon	

Pre heat the oven to 150°C/ 300°F/Gas 2. You will need a 23cm/9 inch square shallow ovenproof dish of about 2 Lt/3½pt capacity.

1   Peel the beetroot. Chop half of it into small ½cm/¼in cubes and coarsely grate the other half.

2   Bring the vegetable stock to the boil and leave it simmering. Put the oven proof dish into the oven to warm.

3   Lightly sauté the chopped onion in the butter for a couple of

minutes. Add the rice with the crushed garlic, cayenne pepper and the lemon zest. Stir until the rice is coated with the butter, then add the grated beetroot. Pour on about 1Lt/2 pints of the vegetable stock. Bring everything to the boil and give it a good stir.

4   Now transfer the rice and stock into the oven proof dish. Stir it once and put it uncovered on the middle of the oven. Cook it for 20 minutes.

5   Take the risotto out of the oven and stir in the rest of the vegetable stock, the rest of the beetroot and the grated parmesan or pecorino. Put it back into the oven for 20 minutes. The rice should be cooked but still have a slight bite to it.

6   Stir in the lemon juice and sprinkle on the chopped herbs and crumbled cheese.

Serve with a green salad, steamed broccoli or French beans.

Broccoli Risotto Torte

This is a savoury 'cake' that is served cut into wedges. It can be eaten hot or cold and needs only a salad as an accompaniment. You can make the torte with barley, spelt, buckwheat, quinoa or risotto rice. The cake has a softer texture when it is made with rice. This is a good way to 'stretch out' the carbohydrates as the risotto cake will easily serve 8 or more people.

SERVES 8

225g/8oz pearl barley

1.2Lt/2¼ pt vegetable stock

1 large onion peeled and finely chopped

50g/1½oz butter

1 tsp cayenne pepper

450g/1lb broccoli broken into florets

1 large courgette quartered lengthways and chopped into 1cm/½ in chunks

100g/3½oz grated parmesan or pecorino

4 large free range eggs separated

1   Melt the butter in a large pan or saucepan, add the onion and sauté it on a medium heat for about 5 minutes.

2   Add the barley and stir it to coat the grains with the butter. Add the cayenne pepper and the vegetable stock, bring to the boil, cover and simmer on a very low heat for 50 minutes. By this time the barley should be soft and most of the stock will have been absorbed. Take off the lid, give it a good stir, put the lid back on and turn off the heat. Leave the barley to cool a little.

3   Grease a 25cm/10in round deep cake tin, a silicon baking tin is ideal.

4   Pre heat the oven to 180ºC/ 350ºF/Gas 4.

5   Blanch the broccoli in boiling water for 3 minutes. Drain and refresh in cold water.

6   Put the courgette into a microwave bowl, cover and cook on full power for 3 minutes.

7   Whisk the egg whites in a clean, dry bowl until they are stiff and form soft peaks.

8   Add the egg yolks and grated cheese to the barley and mix well. Then stir in the broccoli and courgettes. Add a third of the whisked egg whites to the barley mixture and stir until everything is thoroughly mixed. Now gently fold in the remaining egg whites.

9   Pour the mixture into the cake tin, cover with foil and bake for 45 minutes. Take off the foil, put back into the oven and cook for another 15 minutes.

NOTE: Separating the eggs is optional. It gives the torte a lighter texture but if you are in a hurry don't separate the eggs. Just beat them well and stir them into the barley mixture.

Broad Bean & Almond Pilaf

This can be cooked in advance and reheated when you are ready to serve it. You can use quinoa, basmati rice, pearl barley, spelt or buckwheat to make this.

SERVES 4

200g/7oz basmati rice

400ml/14fl oz water

300g/10½oz frozen broad beans

2 tbsp olive oil

3 medium white onions finely sliced

3 cloves garlic crushed

1 tsp vegetable stock powder

1 tsp cayenne pepper

1 tbsp cumin seeds

3 tbsp raisins

40g/1½ oz flaked almonds

2 tbsp lemon juice

Salt and pepper to taste

Pre heat the oven to 180°C/ 350°F/Gas 4

1   Put the almonds onto a baking try and cook them for 7 to 8 minutes until they are light golden brown.

2   Sauté the onions in the oil over a medium heat for 5 minutes. Add the garlic, cayenne pepper and cumin seeds and cook for 2 – 3 minutes.

3   Stir in the rice and the raisins, add then add the water and vegetable stock powder. Bring to the boil, cover, reduce the heat to very low and cook slowly for 12 minutes. Turn off the heat and leave the lid on the pan while you cook the broad beans.

4   Bring the broad beans to the boil and cook for 6 - 7 minutes. Drain and, if you are inclined to or believe you should, peel them. Add the broad beans to the rice and raisins and stir in the lemon juice. Sprinkle the toasted almonds on top and serve.

Tabbouleh

Tabbouleh is traditionally made with bulgar wheat but you can also use quinoa or couscous. This recipe uses coarse bulgar wheat and this needs cooking. If you use fine or medium bulgar wheat all you need to do is soak it in boiling water for 10 minutes. Serve the Tabbouleh on its own or with cannellini bean pate or Tahini. Recipes for these are in the Pates Dips and Sauces section.

SERVES 4

200g/7oz coarse bulgar wheat
400ml/14fl oz water
1 tsp vegetable stock powder
500g/1lb 2oz chopped ripe tomatoes
Small bunch flat leaf parsley
finely chopped
55g/2oz fresh coriander or mint finely
chopped

1 telegraph cucumber peeled, de-seeded
and finely chopped
4 tbsp olive oil
Salt and pepper to taste

1   Bring the water and vegetable stock powder to the boil. Add the bulgar wheat and bring it back to the boil. Turn the heat to low, cover and leave it to cook very gently for 10 minutes. Turn off the heat and leave it to stand covered for at least 15 minutes before removing the lid.

2   When the bulgar wheat is cool stir in the tomatoes, cucumber, parsley, mint and olive oil and season to taste.

You can store the Tabbouleh in the fridge for up to 2 days.

Quinoa, Beetroot & Cucumber Salad
A simple salad that goes really well with hot and cold fish.

SERVES 4

100g/3½oz quinoa
Just under 300ml/10 fl oz water
500g/1lb 2oz packet of cooked beetroot
Half a medium red onion finely chopped
½ telegraph cucumber
3 – 4 heaped tsp grated horseradish
Juice of a lemon

1 tbsp olive oil
1 tbsp finely chopped fresh dill
1 tbsp finely chopped capers
50g/1¾oz packet baby salad leaves or rocket

1 Cook the quinoa and leave it to cool while you prepare the rest of the ingredients.

2 Mix the horseradish with the lemon juice and olive oil in a jam jar. Put on the lid and give it a good shake.

3 Peel the cucumber, cut it in half lengthways and remove the seeds. Chop it into small 5mm/¼ in dice.

4 Rinse and dry the beetroot and cut it into small 5mm/¼ in dice.

5 Add the chopped red onion, the cucumber and the horseradish and lemon juice dressing to the diced beetroot. Stir this into the quinoa then add the capers and the chopped dill.

Serve with a salad of baby leaves.

Quinoa, Avocado, Feta & Tomato Salad

You can use fresh or oven dried tomatoes to make this. The oven dried tomatoes give the salad a more intense flavour. You will find the recipe for oven dried tomatoes in the Hot and Cold Salads section.

SERVES 4

100g/3½oz quinoa

Just under 300ml/10 fl oz water

3 large ripe avocados

200g/7oz feta cut into

5mm/¼ in dice

400g/14oz can red beans drained and rinsed

Small bunch chives finely sliced

16 – 20 oven dried tomatoes cut into quarters

30g/1oz rocket or watercress

2 tbsp lemon or lime juice

1   Wash the quinoa and drain it. Put it into a saucepan, bring it to the boil, cover with a tight fitting lid and reduce to a very low heat. Leave it to cook for 25 – 30 minutes. When it has finished cooking leave it to stand for at least half an hour before taking off the lid.

Alternatively microwave the quinoa following the instructions at the beginning of this section.

2   Cut the avocados in half and remove the stone using a small spoon. Peel them, cut them into 1 cm/½ in dice and cover them with the lemon or lime juice.

3   When the quinoa is cold mix everything together in a large bowl.

Soba Noodle Salad

This is one of those bright fragrant salads that is more vegetables than noodles. It tastes delicious and will keep for up to 2 days in the fridge. You can use rice or soba noodles to make this. If you are avoiding wheat and want to use soba noodles check the label to make sure that they are 100% buckwheat.

You can eat this salad on its own or with fish, seafood or burgers. You can use any combination of vegetables to add to the noodles. Courgettes, baby sweetcorn, mange tout and broccoli work just as well as the vegetables listed here. The list of ingredients in the dressing is long but the recipe is actually easy to make.

SERVES 4 – 6

250g/9 oz soba noodles

2 tsp sesame oil

1 telegraph cucumber peeled, de-seeded and cut into thin batons

2 small carrots, peeled

1 red pepper de-seeded and very finely sliced into rings

100g/4 oz mange tout, cut in half lengthways

50g/1¾oz bean sprouts washed and dried

6 spring onions

2 tbsp toasted sesame seeds

For the dressing:

50ml/2fl oz rice vinegar

50ml/2fl oz Thai fish sauce

2 tsp sugar

125ml/4 fl oz water

1 clove garlic crushed

1 red birds eye chilli very finely chopped OR 1 tsp Sambol Oelek

1 – 2 tbsp finely grated ginger

1 tbsp finely chopped coriander

1 tbsp finely chopped fresh mint

Grated zest of 1 lime

Juice of 2 limes

1   You will need to cook the noodles in line with the instructions on the packet. Usually this means putting them into boiling water, reducing the heat and simmering them for between 5 and 7 minutes. Drain the noodles and refresh them by rinsing them under cold water until all of the starch is removed. Drain them and stir in the sesame oil and sesame seeds. The oil will prevent the

noodles from sticking together.

2   Put the mange tout into a microwave bowl with 3 tablespoons of water. Cover and cook on full power for 3 minutes. Drain and refresh them in cold water.

3   Use a potato peeler to cut the carrots into thin ribbons.

4   Cut the spring onions into matchstick size pieces.

5   To make the dressing. Put all the ingredients into a jar with a lid and give them a good shake to thoroughly mix them.

6   To assemble the salad put all the ingredients together in a large bowl and stir in about a quarter of the dressing. Serve the rest of the dressing in a separate bowl.

Cauliflower, Nut Butter & Miso Noodles

A simple recipe that combines cauliflower and broccoli with noodles, almond butter and miso. Most supermarkets now stock miso, failing this you can buy it on line. You can use any type of broccoli or sprouting kale to make this. The combination of the green broccoli, brown noodles and the white cauliflower looks very attractive.

SERVES 4

450g/1lb cauliflower broken into small florets

900g/2lb broccoli broken into small florets

150g/5½ oz soba noodles

1 tbsp olive oil

30g/1oz toasted flaked almonds

4 spring onions

1 red chilli very finely sliced OR some finely sliced Ramiro pepper

3 tbsp almond butter

1 tbsp white miso paste

Juice and finely grated zest of 1 lime

6 tbsp water

1   Make the almond dressing by mixing the almond butter, miso and lime zest and lime juice together and then slowly whisking in the water until you have a creamy sauce. You can use a hand blender to do this.

2   Cook the noodles in line with the instructions on the packet. Usually this means simmering them for between 5 and 7 minutes. Drain them and stir in the olive oil and the almond dressing.

3   Cook the broccoli and cauliflower in separate saucepans for 3 minutes. They need to be slightly 'al dente'. Drain them, put them into a large bowl or saucepan and stir in the cooked noodles and half of the dressing.. Serve garnished with the toasted almonds, spring onions and sliced chilli or pepper and the remaining dressing in a separate bowl.

Salmon & Rice Noodle Rolls

A good way of making an assortment of vegetables and some cooked salmon or trout into a quick meal.

SERVES 4

12 thin rice paper pancakes

60g/2¼oz pea sprouts or mustard cress

50g/1¾oz rice vermicelli

2 large ripe avocados

½ telegraph cucumber peeled, de-seeded and cut into thin batons

Small bunch of chives finely chopped

2 tbsp lemon juice

1 heaped tsp grated horseradish

50ml/2fl oz fromage frais

2 tsp finely chopped fresh dill

2 tsp finely grated lemon or lime zest

150g/5½oz cooked salmon, skinned, boned and flaked

100g/3½oz cooked prawns

1   Place the rice vermicelli in a heatproof bowl, cover them with boiling water and leave them to soak until they are just tender. This usually takes between 3 and 5 minutes. Drain them, refresh them in cold water and leave them draining in a sieve while you prepare the other ingredients.

2   Mix together the fromage frais, horseradish, lemon or lime zest, chives and chopped dill.

3   Cut the avocados in half and remove the stone using a small spoon. Peel them, slice them thinly and cover them with the lemon juice.

4   Put the rice noodles into a large bowl and stir in the fromage frais mixture, the cucumber, peas sprouts, prawns and salmon.

5   Spread a clean tea towel onto your work surface. Put some hand hot water into a wide bowl and place 1 sheet of the rice paper pancakes in to soak until it is just softened and flexible. This usually takes about 20 seconds. Lift it out carefully and place it onto tea towel.

6   Put 2 tbsp of the rice noodle mixture on the edge of the pancake nearest you and put some slices of avocado on top. Fold in the 2 sides, then the bottom edge so that it covers the filling. Roll the pancake up holding the filling firmly.

7   Repeat with the remaining rice paper pancakes.

Cover with cling film or foil until you are ready to serve.

PASTA, GNOCCHI & PIZZA

Pasta, Pizza and Gnocchi are to most of us synonymous with 'fast food' and, despite their relatively healthy Mediterranean origins, in the western diet, they have evolved into a notoriously unhealthy food.

Unless you buy the 'free from' brands you find in supermarkets pasta is made from highly refined wheat and refined wheat is a high glycemic index, highly inflammatory food. So where does pasta and pizza fit into a diet to treat gout and inflammation? Simply by combining it with ingredients that are anti-inflammatory the pro-inflammatory effect can be balanced out; anchovies, sardines, salmon, onion, garlic and spinach are all powerful anti-inflammatory foods.

Interestingly most pasta has a medium to low glycaemic index. If you cook the pasta until it is 'al dente' and then leave it to cool to room temperature it's glycaemic index reduces further because the starch molecules 'rearrange' themselves during the cooling process and become more resistant to being digested. If you reheat the pasta with a sauce and some vegetables it's glycemic index is reduced even more. Provided it is rinsed and cooled quickly after you have cooked it you can keep cooked pasta in a covered container in the fridge for up to 3 days.

Whole wheat pasta contains less iron and more fibre than pasta made from refined white flour. Because of this when you eat whole wheat pasta you feel fuller for longer. However, as most of the following pasta recipes are packed full of the vegetables and fibre that also give you the 'full' feeling, whether you use whole wheat or white pasta is a matter of personal choice.

To most of us Pizza means bread dough, usually thick but sometimes thin, with some form of topping and cheese. Usually a Pizza is more 'bread' than topping and often more 'cheese' than topping. Commercial Pizza especially, with far too much salt and sugar added, it is not a particularly healthy food, but this is not necessarily the way 'Pizza' is made in Mediterranean countries.

There are many different types of 'Pizza' and most of them are loaded with herbs and spices and these go some way to mitigating the inflammatory effect of the wheat. Almost without exception they also have more 'topping' than base.

Like pasta and pizza, gnocchi are synonymous with starchy carbohydrates. Potatoes and semolina usually come to mind and gnocchi are often made with full fat cream cheese. The following recipes use silken tofu instead of the cream cheese as this is a much healthier protein rich alternative and you do not have to use potatoes and semolina either.

Making gnocchi takes time but it is worth the effort as home made gnocchi tastes so much better than the gnocchi you buy in packets in the supermarket. Once you have made the gnocchi you can cook them in many different ways.

All types of gnocchi freeze well and because of this they are one of the store cupboard staples that are worth making in large quantities and storing in the freezer as your own supply of 'fast food'. The Japanese panko breadcrumbs used in the recipes for gnocchi is not authentic and yes, the breadcrumbs are inflammatory, but they are used in small amounts and they give the gnocchi a light fluffy texture. If you are avoiding wheat use polenta instead. The gnocchi will not be quite as fluffy but they will still be good to eat.

CONTENTS

Cauliflower, Tomato & Anchovy Pasta

This is a quick and easy dish that you can prepare in advance and heat up in the microwave at the last minute. You can use any type of 'large' non spaghetti like pasta to make this. Adjust the amount of garlic and chilli you use to suit your taste. If you add some butter beans or cannellini beans you can make this into a really substantial meal that will feed up to 6 people. You will find the recipe for Tapenade in the Herbs and Spices section.

SERVES 4 - 6

1 large cauliflower

200g/7oz cherry tomatoes cut in half

4 cloves garlic crushed

1 red chilli finely chopped OR 1 tsp Sambol Oelek or chilli paste

50g/1¾oz tin anchovy fillets in olive oil

3 tbsp capers

16 - 20 salted black olives stones removed and cut in half

3 tbsp finely sliced basil

150g/5½oz orchietta, large pasta shells or thick pasta tubes

Crushed black pepper (optional)

400g/14 oz tine butter beans or cannellini beans drained and rinsed

2 tbsp lightly toasted pine nuts

4 tbsp finely grated parmesan or pecorino

1 tbsp black olive tapenade (optional)

2 tbsp olive oil (optional)

1   Cook the pasta in line with the instructions on the packet. Just make sure it is 'al dente' still has some bite when you have finished cooking it. Put it to one side while you make the rest of the dish.

2   If you are using it, mix the tapenade with the olive oil.

3   Remove the outside leaves from the cauliflower and break the inside into small florets about the size of your thumb. Cook these for about 3 minutes until they are just tender. Drain, reserving about 50ml/2 fl oz of the cooking liquid and put to one side.

4   Drain the oil from the anchovies into a large saucepan or wok and cut the anchovies into 1 cm/½ in pieces.

5   Heat the oil from the anchovies over a medium heat and add the
    garlic and the chilli. Because of the fluid in it the oil will spit a little.
    Cook the garlic and chilli for 2 – 3 minutes but do not let it brown.

6   Stir in the capers, the olives and tomatoes and the reserved
    cooking liquid from the cauliflower. Now stir in the cooked pasta,
    the cauliflower and, if you are using them, the beans. Cover and
    cook slowly just long enough to heat through.

7   Just before serving stir in half of the grated parmesan or pecorino
    and sprinkle on the shredded basil and toasted pine nuts.

    Serve the rest of the parmesan and the black olive tapenade in
    separate bowls.

Sardine Pasta

*This is one concession to 'pasta and some sauce' as opposed to
'vegetables, sauce and some pasta'. It is one of the quickest and easiest
pasta dishes you can make and, because of the oily fish and tomato, it
is good, anti-inflammatory food. You can use any type of tinned oily
fish to make this. Just make sure you buy fish that is canned in olive oil
and try to buy fish fillets as opposed to whole fish, that way you do not
have to remove the bones.*

SERVES 4

200g/7oz linguine or spaghetti

2 x 120g/4¼ oz tins sardine fillets in
olive oil

1 medium red onion finely chopped

4 tbsp tomato purée

3 tbsp capers

4 cloves garlic crushed

1 small red chilli finely chopped or 1 tsp
Sambol Oelek or chilli paste

1 tbsp Thai fish sauce OR 1 tsp anchovy
paste

2 tbsp water

3 tbsp finely grated parmesan

1   Cook the pasta in line with the instructions on the packet. Just
    make sure it is 'al dente' and still has some bite when you have
    finished cooking it. Drain it, reserving a couple of tablespoons of
    the cooking liquid for later.

2   Drain the oil from the sardines into a large saucepan and heat it
    over a medium heat. Add the red onion, garlic, chilli and tomato
    purée. Cook for 5 minutes.

3   Flake the sardines and stir them in with the capers. Then add the
    Thai fish sauce or anchovy paste and the water. Now stir in the
    cooked pasta. Cover and cook slowly to heat the pasta through.

4   Just before serving stir in half of the grated parmesan. Serve with a
    green salad and the rest of the parmesan in a separate bowl.

Salmon Pasta & Red Pepper Sauce

Ideally the red peppers should be roasted and then peeled before being blended into the yoghurt. However, the recipe works just as well if the peppers are sautéed with half a teaspoon of smoked paprika. This recipe uses Rigatoni but you can use any type of large, chunky pasta. You can make this in advance and heat it through when you are ready to eat it.

SERVES 4

700g/1 lb 9oz salmon
3 large red peppers
3 tbsp olive oil
1 medium white or red onion roughly chopped
1 clove garlic crushed (optional)
1 tsp Sambol Oelek or chilli paste
90ml/3 fl oz dry white wine or water

½ tsp smoked paprika
125ml/4 fl oz natural unsweetened Greek style yoghurt
Salt and pepper to taste
200g/7oz Rigatoni
70g/2½oz baby spinach
Finely chopped parsley or chervil to garnish

1   Skin and bone the salmon and cut it into 2cm/¾ in pieces.

2   Cut the peppers in half, de-seed them and slice them thinly.

3   Heat 1 tbsp of the olive oil in a saucepan on a fairly high heat and add the peppers. Stir fry for 5 minutes to bring out the flavour of the peppers but don't let them brown.

4   Take out half of the peppers and put them to one side. Add the chopped onion and add the crushed garlic. Turn down the heat, stir for a minute and then add the white wine or water. Bring to the boil, cover, reduce the heat and simmer for 15 minutes. Turn off the heat and leave the peppers in the saucepan.

5   Cook the pasta in line with the instructions on the packet. Just make sure it is 'al dente' and still has some bite when you have finished cooking it. Stir in the baby spinach and leave the spinach to wilt for a minute before you drain the pasta. Stir the reserved

peppers and a tablespoon of olive oil into the drained pasta to prevent it sticking together.

6   While the pasta is cooking, heat the remaining oil over a medium heat in a non stick frying pan. Add the salmon and cook for 5 minutes until it is just set.

7   Add the yoghurt to the peppers in the saucepan and use a hand blender to blend the peppers into a thick sauce. Mix a quarter of this into the pasta, spinach and peppers.

8   Add the cooked salmon to the rest of the pepper sauce and gently stir it in. Serve the pasta and wilted spinach with the salmon and red pepper sauce on top.

Pasta a Faglio

This is an adaptation of a classic Italian dish that is more like a stew than a soup. The authentic dish uses dried borlotti beans that are soaked overnight before being cooked. Canned beans are much quicker. You can cook the pasta in advance and add it to the stew at the last minute.

SERVES 6

2 x 400g/14 ox can of borlotti beans drained and rinsed

1 large onion finely sliced

3 tbsp olive oil

1 large leek finely sliced

2 large carrots peeled and finely chopped

2 sticks celery finely chopped

1 large potato peeled and chopped into 1cm/½ in dice

4 cloves of garlic crushed

600ml/20fl oz (1pt) vegetable stock

½ tsp dried thyme

½ tsp dried rosemary

½ tsp dried sage

200g/7oz conchiglie or small pasta shells

10 large tomatoes each cut into 8 pieces

2 tbsp tomato purée

Salt and ground black pepper

Finely grated parmesan and finely Chopped parsley or chervil to serve

1   Heat the olive oil in a large saucepan and add the sliced onions, leeks, potatoes and carrots. Sauté for 5 minutes and then add the garlic, thyme, rosemary and sage.

2   Stir in the vegetable stock, the tomato purée and the borlotti beans. Bring to the boil, reduce the heat, cover and leave the 'stew' simmering while you cook the pasta.

3   Add the pasta to a large saucepan of boiling water. Cook for 7 to 8 minutes until it is just cooked, then drain it.

4   Add the pasta to the bean stew and stir in the tomatoes. Scatter some chopped parsley and grated parmesan over the top and serve the rest of the parmesan in a separate bowl.

Courgette & Red Pepper Lasagne

*Ready to use lasagne makes lasagne fairly quick and easy to make.
Even though the instructions on the packet do not tell you to, pre-
soaking the sheets of lasagne while you prepare the filling improves the
texture. You will need a 5cm/2 in deep large ovenproof dish or casserole
that takes 3 sheets of lasagne across the base to make this. A dish that
is 24cm x 20 cm or 10 in x 8 in is ideal. You will find the recipe for basil
pesto in the Herbs and Spices section.*

SERVES 6

9 sheets ready to use lasagne

6 spring onions finely sliced

1 clove garlic crushed (optional)

400g/14 oz can chopped tomatoes

3 tbsp tomato purée

1 tsp cayenne pepper

4 tbsp fromage frais or natural
unsweetened yoghurt

3 large free range eggs

3 tbsp finely grated parmesan.

2 large red peppers

400g/14 oz courgettes thinly sliced

For the topping:

350g/12oz packet silken tofu

100ml/3½ fl oz milk

1 large free range egg

60g/2¼oz basil pesto

3 tbsp finely grated parmesan

1 Pre heat the oven to 200ºC/ 400ºF/Gas 5 and grease the baking
   dish.

2 Put the sheets of lasagne into a large shallow bowl and cover them
   with hot water. Leave them to soak while you prepare the filling.

3 Cut the red peppers into quarters and remove the seeds. Put them
   onto a baking tray lined with non stick foil and roast them for 20
   to 25 minutes. Tip them into a bowl and cover them with cling film.

4 Put the sliced courgette into a microwave bowl, cover and cook for
   3 minutes until it is just beginning to soften.

5 Whisk the eggs, tomato purée, cayenne pepper, fromage frais and
   parmesan together. Stir in the spring onions, the copped tomatoes

and the garlic. If there is any fluid in the bowl with the courgettes drain this off and stir this in as well.

6   When the peppers are cool enough to handle remove the cling film and peel off the skin. You do not need to remove all of the skin, but make sure you take off any skin that looks black and charred. Keep any oil that is in the bowl.

7   Drain the sheets of lasagne. Put 3 sheets of the lasagne in a layer on the bottom of the ovenproof dish. Spoon on a third of the tomato mixture. On top of this arrange the courgettes is an even layer and then spoon on another third of the tomato mixture on top.

8   Put 3 sheets of lasagne on top of this and then add the roasted red peppers. Pour on any oil that is in the bowl. Spoon on the last of the tomato mixture and put the last 3 sheets of lasagne on top.

9   Use a hand blender to mix the tofu with the pesto, egg, milk and 2 tablespoons of the grated parmesan. Pour this on top. Cover with foil and bake for 30 minutes at 200°C/ 400°F/Gas 5. Remove the foil and sprinkle on the remaining tablespoon of grated parmesan and cook for another 10 minutes.

Spinach & Mushroom Lasagne

Use fresh or frozen leaf spinach or if you can get it Swiss chard.

SERVES 4

9 sheets pre-cooked lasagne

400g /14 oz cooked spinach or
Swiss chard

3 tbsp pine nuts lightly toasted

200g /7oz ricotta or crumbled feta

3 spring onions finely sliced

¼ tsp grated nutmeg

225g/8 oz chestnut mushrooms

2 tbsp olive oil

1 tsp garlic granules

1 tsp ground coriander

1 tsp sesame oil

For the topping:

400ml/14fl oz fromage frais or natural
unsweetened yoghurt

100ml/3½ fl oz milk

1 large free range egg

3 tbsp finely grated parmesan

1   Put the sheets of lasagne into a large shallow bowl and cover them
    with hot water. Leave them to soak while you prepare the filling.

2   Heat the olive oil in a saucepan, add the mushrooms and sauté
    them over a high heat for 5 minutes. Stir them every minute to
    prevent them sticking.

3   Stir in the garlic granules and ground coriander, reduce the heat to
    medium, cover and cook for another 5 minutes. Stir in the sesame
    oil, replace the lid and remove from the heat.

    Pre heat the oven to 200°C/ 400°F/Gas 5

4   Squeeze the spinach or chard to make sure it is dry and mix it with
    the toasted pine nuts, chopped spring onions, grated nutmeg and
    the ricotta or crumbled feta.

5   Use a hand blender to mix the fromage frais with the egg, milk and
    2 tablespoons of the grated parmesan.

6   Drain the sheets of lasagne.

7   Put 3 sheets of the lasagne in a layer on the bottom of the
    ovenproof dish. Spoon on a third of the fromage frais, milk and
    egg mixture. On top of this arrange the spinach in an even layer.

8   Put 3 sheets of lasagne on top of this and then add the
    mushrooms. Pour on any juice that is in the pan with the
    mushrooms. Put the last 3 sheets of lasagne on top.

9   Pour the rest of the fromage frais and egg mixture on top. Cover
    with foil and bake for 30 minutes at 200°C/ 400°F/Gas 5. Remove
    the foil and sprinkle on the remaining tablespoon of grated
    parmesan and cook for another 10 minutes.

Vegetable Gnocchi with Tandoori Spices

You can use this recipe for vegetable gnocchi in different ways and
serve it with many different sauces. This recipe bakes the gnocchi with
tandoori spices. The recipe uses chopped green garlic which you can
buy frozen from Asian supermarkets. Use a teaspoon of garlic granules
and a tablespoon of sliced spring onions if you do not have any. If you
are cooking all of the gnocchi at the same time you will need to double
the amount of tandoori spice mixture.

Makes about 30 gnocchi
350g/12oz packet of silken tofu
1 free range egg
100g/3½oz grated carrot
100g/3½oz grated courgette
50g/1¾oz cooked peas
2 tbsp finely chopped parsley OR
30g/1oz ready made gremolata
Finely grated zest of ½ lemon
3 tbsp toasted sesame seeds
50g/1¾oz Japanese panko breadcrumbs
60g/2¼oz fine oatmeal
2 tbsp chopped green garlic

For the tandoori spices:
1 tbsp finely grated ginger
1 tbsp crushed garlic
½ tsp chilli powder OR 1 tsp Sambol Oelek
1 tsp turmeric
1 tbsp ground cumin
2 tbsp olive oil
2 tbsp lemon juice
To serve:
½ red onion finely chopped
300g/10½oz broccoli florets

1   Put the grated carrots and courgettes into a microwave bowl, cover
    and cook on full power 3 minutes. Leave them to cool while you
    prepare the other ingredients.

2   Put the tofu, egg, parsley, lemon zest and oatmeal into a bowl and
    mix with a hand blender until the mixture is smooth.

3   When the carrots and courgettes have cooled down, add them to
    the tofu and egg mixture with the sesame seeds, and breadcrumbs
    and mix well. Do not be alarmed if at this stage the mixture is a
    quite soft. The egg, breadcrumbs and oatmeal will hold the

gnocchi together as soon as they are cooked. Cover and put the mixture in the fridge for several hours or even better, overnight.

4   Spread a pastry board with flour or fine polenta and form spoonfuls of the mixture into small balls about the size of a walnut. Roll them in flour or polenta and lay them out on a floured tray.

5   Bring a large pan of slightly salted water to the boil, then turn it down to a steady simmer. You will need to cook the gnocchi in batches as they need plenty of room, so have a tray lined with a towel or some kitchen paper ready for them.

6   Gently lower 6 to 7 gnocchi into the water and leave them to simmer gently. When they rise to the surface, which will be in about 4 to 6 minutes, they are ready. They will disintegrate if you leave them too long so take them out with a perforated spoon and leave them to drain while you cook the rest. At this stage you can either carry on with the recipe or transfer the gnocchi to a tray lined with cling film or non stick foil and open freeze them in a single layer before packaging them up.

7   To cook the gnocchi heat the oven to 200°C/ 400°F/Gas 5.

8   Mix together the tandoori spices in a large bowl and stir in the gnocchi until they are covered with the spice mixture. Leave them to marinade while the oven heats up. Put the gnocchi onto a non stick baking tray or a baking tray lined with non stick foil. Bake them for 20 minutes turning them once.

9   Cook the broccoli in boiling water for 3 minutes. Before draining it pour 150ml/5 fl oz of the cooking water into a small saucepan. Add the chopped red onion, a teaspoon of vegetable stock powder and the remains of the tandoori marinade. Bring to the boil and simmer for 5 minutes and then pour over the broccoli. Arrange the gnocchi on top and serve.

Pumpkin Gnocchi with Rocket Pesto

You can serve the gnocchi with a variety of different sauces. If you have some frozen gnocchi, frozen pesto and a bag of ready to eat rocket or baby spinach you have a very quick meal.

Makes a lot

500g/1lb 2oz cooked pumpkin or butternut squash

150g/5½oz fine polenta

1 large free range egg

Salt and crushed black pepper

85g/3oz quark or ricotta or any other low fat cream cheese

1 tsp dried sage

½ tsp grated nutmeg

For the rocket pesto:

100g/3½oz rocket

50g/1¾oz grated parmesan

½ tsp grain mustard

1 tsp Sambol Oelek or chilli paste

Juice ½ lemon

1 tbsp caper vinegar OR white wine vinegar

50g/1¾oz ground almonds

4 tbsp olive oil

Crushed garlic to taste

To serve

30g/1oz rocket

2 tbsp toasted pine nuts

2 tbsp finely grated parmesan.

1   Roughly chop the cooked pumpkin or butternut squash and put it into a large bowl. Blend it with a hand blender until it is smooth.

2   Add the remaining ingredients, season to taste and mix well. If the mixture looks too wet add a tablespoon of Japanese panko breadcrumbs. Cover and put the mixture in the fridge for several hours or overnight

3   To make the rocket pesto. Wash and dry the rocket and remove any tough leaves. Put everything into a food processor and blend until fully mixed.

4   To make the gnocchi, spread a pastry board with flour and form spoonfuls of the mixture into small croquettes about the size of a cork. Roll them in flour and lay them out on a floured tray.

5   Bring a large pan of slightly salted water to the boil, then turn it down to a steady simmer. You will need to cook the gnocchi in batches as they need plenty of room, so have a tray lined with a clean towel or some kitchen paper ready for them.

6   Using a perforated draining spoon gently lower 8 to 10 gnocchi into the water. When they rise to the top, which will be in about 5 to 8 minutes, they are ready. They will disintegrate if you leave them too long so take them out with the perforated spoon and leave them to drain while you cook the rest.

7   At this stage you can freeze the gnocchi or use them in the recipe.

8   To serve the gnocchi, fill a large pan with water, bring it to the boil and turn down the heat to leave the water just simmering. Put the gnocchi in and leave them gently simmering for a couple of minutes to heat through, take them out with a perforated spoon. Stir in the pesto, the toasted pine nuts and the rocket and sprinkle over the parmesan.

Spinach Gnocchi with Tomato Sauce

The tomato sauce used in this recipe is included in the section on sauces. The sauce tastes delicious and it is worth making in large quantities, without the garlic, and storing it in the freezer. With frozen tomato sauce, frozen gnocchi and some salad you have a very quick meal, your own fast food.

Makes a lot
350g/12oz cooked spinach
350g/12oz silken tofu
100g/3½oz finely grated parmesan
or pecorino
1 large free range egg and 1 egg yolk
6 tbsp potato flour or fine polenta
3 tbsp Japanese panko bread crumbs OR
polenta
¼ tsp grated nutmeg
salt and pepper

Rich Tomato Sauce
1 large red onion finely chopped
3 tbsp olive oil

2 400g/14 oz cans of chopped tomatoes
3 tbsp tomato purée
2 tsp vegetable stock powder
1 tbsp anchovy paste
6 cloves garlic finely sliced
1 tbsp red wine vinegar
1 tbsp sugar
20 salted black olives, stones removed and
cut into quarters
2 tbsp finely shredded basil
2 tbsp finely grated parmesan

1   Put the tofu, spinach, egg and egg yolk, potato flour, grated parmesan and grated nutmeg into a bowl and mix with a hand blender until the mixture is smooth. Stir in the breadcrumbs and season to taste.

2   Cover and put the mixture in the fridge for several hours or overnight.

3   To make the tomato sauce. Sauté the onion and sliced garlic in the oil for 10 minutes, stirring a couple of times. Don't let the onion or garlic brown. Add the chopped tomatoes, vegetable stock powder,

tomato purée, anchovy paste, red wine vinegar and sugar. Cover
and leave to simmer over a low heat.

4   Spread a pastry board with flour and form spoonfuls of the
gnocchi mixture into small balls or little croquettes about the size
of a cork. Roll them in flour and lay them out on a floured tray.

5   Bring a large pan of slightly salted water to the boil, then turn it
down to a steady simmer. You will need to cook the gnocchi in
batches as they need plenty of room, so have a tray lined with a
clean towel or some kitchen paper ready for them.

6   Using a perforated draining spoon gently lower 8 to 10 gnocchi
into the water. When they rise to the top, which will be in about 5
to 8 minutes, they are ready. They will disintegrate if you leave
them too long so take them out with the perforated spoon and
leave them to drain on the tray while you cook the rest.

At this stage you can either carry on with the recipe or transfer
them to a tray lined with cling film or non stick foil and open
freeze them in a single layer before packaging them up.

7   To cook the gnocchi heat the oven to 180°C/ 350°F/Gas 4

8   Add half of the shredded basil and black olives to the tomato
sauce and turn off the heat. Put the gnocchi into an oven proof
dish and pour over the tomato sauce. Bake, uncovered for 15
minutes. Sprinkle with the remaining basil and grated parmesan
before serving.

Socca

Socca is a thin savoury pancake that is made from chickpea flour (gram flour), olive oil and water. It's origin is in the area around Nice in the South of France. The southern Italians have a similar type of pancake which they call Farinatta. Many supermarkets now sell gram flour, which incidentally is gluten free, but you may need to hunt it down in an Asian supermarket or buy it online.

You can eat Socca and Farinatta on its own as a savoury egg free 'pancake', as an alternative to bread, pancakes and drop scones or use it as a base for pizzas and vegetable dishes. Traditional Socca is simple in terms of its flavour but you can vary it's flavour by adding herbs and spices.

The following recipe is sufficient to make one 24cm/10 in Socca. You can make the Socca in a non stick frying pan, a cast iron pan or a silicon sponge or cake tin. The Socca can be eaten hot or cold.

SERVES 4

For the Socca
120g/4¼ oz chickpea/gram flour sieved
230ml/8 fl oz tepid water
Juice ½ lemon
1 - 2 crushed cloves of garlic
½ tsp ground cumin
½ tsp chilli flakes

½ tsp ground turmeric
Finely grated zest of ½ lemon
4 tbsp olive oil + 1 tbsp olive oil for cooking

1   Sieve the chickpea flour as it tends to go a bit lumpy.

2   Put all of the ingredients into a bowl and whisk well until you have a smooth, creamy batter. Cover and leave in a warm room for at least 1 hour.

Pre heat the oven to 240°C/ 500°F/Gas 7

3   The batter needs to be put into a hot pan so put the pan into the oven to heat up. If you are using a silicon baking tin put it onto a baking sheet before putting it into the oven as this will make it easier to handle.

4   Whisk the batter. Take the pan out of the oven and put in the remaining 1 tbsp olive oil. Swirl it around to coat the base of the pan. Pour in the batter and put the pan back into the oven and cook for 8 to 10 minutes. By this time the Socca should have shrunk away from the sides of the pan.

Variations:

Olive and Parsley: To the basic Socca mix add 2 tbsp chopped black olives, 2 tbsp chopped parsley and 2 tbsp finely chopped red onions

Lime and Coriander: Omit the lemon juice and lemon zest and add the finely grated zest and juice of one lime plus 3 tbsp finely chopped coriander

Rosemary and Onion: Add 2 tsp dried rosemary and 70g/2½ oz finely grated white onion.

Socca with Shallot Chutney & Tomato

One of the traditional ways of eating Socca is with sliced fresh tomatoes and black olives. The shallot chutney is an optional extra.

SERVES 4

For the chutney
4 banana shallots cut in half and
finely sliced
2 tbsp olive oil
4 large ripe vine tomatoes finely sliced
2 tbsp tomato purée
2 tsp ground cumin
3 tbsp red or white wine vinegar
Salt and pepper to taste

For the Socca
A basic 24cm/10 in Socca made
from 120g/4 oz of chickpea flour
For the topping:
450g/1lb ripe vine tomatoes thinly sliced
3 tbsp capers or caper berries
3 tbsp shredded basil
1 tbsp olive oil

1 To make the chutney. Heat the olive oil and sauté the shallots over a medium heat for 5 minutes. Add the ground cumin, tomatoes, tomato purée and wine vinegar, bring to the boil, reduce the heat, cover and simmer for 15 minutes.

2 Season the chutney to taste and use a hand blender to lightly blend it. The chutney needs to be mixed together but not 'mushed'

3 Cook the Socca. Reduce the oven temperature to 220°C/ 450°F/Gas 6.

4 Put the Socca onto an ovenproof plate and spread on the shallot chutney. Arrange the sliced tomatoes and capers on top and cook for 10 – 15 minutes until the tomatoes are cooked.

5 Sprinkle on the basil and serve with a green salad.

Pizza with Onions & Anchovies

Not quite the pizza we are used to but just as good, and it is much quicker to make as there is no need to prove the dough or roll out the base. The pizza 'crust' is an adaptation of an 18th Century recipe for soda bread that was made with oatmeal and wholegrain flour.

You can make the pizza base and use any type of topping, with or without tomato and with or without cheese. This recipe uses just onions and olives, a way pizza is often served in Rome. Both the pizza base and the onion confit used as the topping can be made in advance and stored in the fridge. They also freeze well.

SERVES 4

For the pizza base:
60g/2¼oz wholegrain spelt
60g/2¼oz fine oatmeal
1 tsp baking powder
3 tbsp olive oil
250ml/9 fl oz milk

For the topping:
450g/1lb white onions finely sliced
100g/3½oz soft low fat cheese such as Quark or ricotta

Finely grated zest of ½ lemon
Juice of ½ lemon
2 bay leaves
Crushed black pepper
50g/1¾oz tin anchovy fillets in olive oil
24 salted black olives stones removed and cut in half
2 tbsp pine nuts

1   You will need a 24cm/10 in round silicon tin or spring form tin to make this. If you are using an ordinary tin grease it well.

2   First make the onion confit. Drain half of the oil from the anchovies into a saucepan, add the onions and gently sauté them over a medium heat for 5 minutes.

3   Add the bay leaves and lemon zest, cover the saucepan, reduce the heat to low and simmer the onions for 30 – 40 minutes until they are soft. Check them once in a while to make sure they are not

burning, sticking or turning brown. Add a tablespoon of water if you need to.

4   Remove the bay leaves and leave the onions to cool slightly before stirring in the lemon juice and the ricotta.

Pre heat the oven to 200°C/ 400°F/Gas 5

5   To make the pizza base. Mix the spelt, fine oatmeal and baking powder together.

6   Whisk the olive oil into the milk.

7   Add the milk and oil to the flour. It will start bubbling as soon as the milk is added to the flour so mix it quickly to form a batter and pour it into the baking tin. Put it into the oven straight away and bake for 12 minutes. By this time it should be lightly browned and firm to the touch. Turn it over and put it back into the oven for 3 minutes to dry off the base.

8   To assemble the pizza, put the pizza base onto an ovenproof plate or baking tray and spoon on the onion mixture. Arrange the black olives and anchovies on top and sprinkle on the pine nuts. Drizzle over the remaining oil from the anchovy fillets. Bake for 10 minutes to heat the topping through.

Cheats Calzone

If you are avoiding gluten this recipe is not for you. If you want a really quick meal every so often you can make this with commercial tortillas from the Supermarket and a commercial sweet chilli sauce. Yes, the commercial sweet chilli sauce will probably contain mono sodium glutamate as well as sugar but it's what you do most of the time not what you do some of the time that matters.

You can use any type of hard cheese, goats or sheep's cheese is very good. Serve the calzone with refried beans and some salad.

Makes 4 small calzone
4 commercial tortillas
4 tbsp sweet chilli sauce
2 ripe avocados
2 tbsp lemon or lime juice
8 tbsp grated cheese

Pre heat the oven to 180°C/ 350°F/Gas 4.

1   Cut the avocados in half and use a small spoon to remove the stone. Peel the avocados and slice them thinly. Drizzle the lemon juice over them to prevent them turning brown.

2   Microwave the tortillas for 30 seconds to make them pliable.

3   Put the tortillas onto a board. Spread a tablespoon of the sweet chilli sauce over one half. Put the slices of one half of an avocado on top and sprinkle on 2 tablespoon of grated cheese Fold the tortilla over to cover the filling.

4   Put the calzone onto a baking tray lined with non stick foil and bake for 10 minutes.

HOT & COLD SALADS

Salads can be a refreshing accompaniment to a main dish or the distinctive centrepiece of a meal. They can be made from cooked as well as raw ingredients and served cold, hot or at room temperature.

Salads are probably the most versatile dishes in the kitchen as they provide endless possibilities of different combinations of colour, flavour and texture. They can usually be put together in minutes and they are very nutritious. With the wide range of ingredients we have available to us today you can enjoy trying out new recipes and experimenting with your own ideas.

Store salad leaves, preferably unwashed, in the fridge and wash and dry them when needed.

CONTENTS

Carrot, Mango & Coriander Salad

This is one of the most weird salads ever, but it tastes absolutely delicious and strangely, it goes extremely well with fish, especially salmon, trout and smoked mackerel. You can serve the salad on its own or add chickpeas or beans to make it into a substantial meal.

Unfortunately its preparation is somewhat labour intensive as it involves a lot of peeling and slicing. If you can obtain one of the sour green mangos that are grown especially for savoury dishes all the better. Otherwise use the most under ripe mango you can find.

SERVES 4

1 very large green under ripe mango

350g/12oz carrots

1 small red onion peeled and finely chopped

3 - 4 tbsp finely chopped coriander OR 30g/1oz ready made coriander pesto

Grated zest of 1 lime

Juice of 1 lime

1 tsp Sambol Oelek or chilli paste

1tbsp rice vinegar

1 tbsp Thai fish sauce

1 preserved lemon

3 tbsp lightly toasted pumpkin and sunflower seeds

1   First make the salad dressing by mixing together the zest and juice of a lime, the Sambol Oelek (you can use more than 1 tsp if you like your food spicy), the rice vinegar, the Thai fish sauce and the chopped coriander or pesto.

2   Cut the stone from the mango. Peel the halves of mango and slice the flesh into thin slices. Now cut each of these thin slices into narrow mandolin strips. Put them into a large bowl and pour on the dressing.

3   Peel the carrots and slice them very thinly along their length. Then cut each long slice into narrow very thin mandolin strips.

4   Add the carrots to the mango in the bowl and give everything a

good stir.

5 Stir in the finely chopped red onion. You can use spring onions if you prefer but the red onion gives the salad a better colour and more intense flavour.

6 Cut the preserved lemon in half, take out the pips and cut it into very small pieces. Stir it into the salad.

7 Lastly add the toasted seeds. You can use more or less toasted seeds according to taste.

8 Cover and leave the salad for at least half an hour for the flavours to develop.

The salad will keep for up to two days if stored in the fridge but the longer you keep it the more the texture will reduce.

Red Cabbage, Bean & Walnut Salad

This is a variation on a traditional red bean and walnut salad from the Caucuses. While in no way authentic, the pickled walnuts give this version of the salad its characteristic flavour. If you are unable to obtain pickled walnuts increase the amount of walnuts and use some Worcestershire Sauce instead of the pickled walnut vinegar.

Serve the salad as an appetiser or as part of a main meal. It works particularly well with savoury cheesecakes.

SERVES 4

½ small red cabbage very finely shredded

1 medium red onion finely sliced

400g/14oz can red beans drained and rinsed

50g/1¾oz finely chopped walnuts

1 pickled walnut finely chopped

2 tbsp walnut oil

2 tbsp pickled walnut vinegar

1 tsp chilli paste or Sambol Oelek

1 clove garlic crushed (optional)

Juice and finely grated zest of a lime

2 tbsp finely chopped coriander OR 1 tbsp ready made coriander pesto

1   Mix together the walnuts, pickled walnuts, vinegar, walnut oil, chilli, lime juice, grated lime zest, crushed garlic and coriander.

2   Mix together the cabbage, red onion and beans, stir in the dressing, cover and chill. The salad will keep for 2 days in a covered container in the fridge.

Oven Dried Tomatoes

Oven dried tomatoes are similar to sun blushed tomatoes. They have a lighter flavour than sun dried tomatoes which can sometime be quite strong. Oven drying is a good way of improving the flavour of tomatoes that have been picked when they are slightly under ripe and they also provide a useful 'store cupboard' source of tomatoes as they freeze extremely well.

The best tomatoes to use are the large 'egg' or 'plum' tomatoes. Failing this use vine ripened tomatoes, the bigger the better. If you can only get your hands on ordinary tomatoes use the second recipe for drying them as this brings out their flavour more. Making oven dried tomatoes is really simple but they do need quite a lot of salt to help in they drying process.

Line your baking trays with foil as this saves on the washing up. Put a grid onto each tray.

Method 1

Pre heat the oven to 120°C/ 250°F/Gas 1

Wash and dry the tomatoes and cut them in half. Arrange them in a single layer on the grids, cut side up.

LIGHTLY sprinkle some sea salt flakes over them and put them uncovered in the oven to cook for about 2 to 3 hours. Open the door every half hour to let out the steam. If the tomatoes are large they may take longer to dry out. They will shrink a lot during the drying process. The tomatoes are ready when the outside is dried and a bit shrivelled but there is still a small amount of moisture inside.

Method 2

Pre heat the oven to 150°C/ 300°F/Gas 2

Wash and dry the tomatoes and cut them in half.

For 2Kg/4 lb 8oz tomatoes you will need to mix together 2 tsp sea salt flakes, 1 tsp garlic granules, ½ tsp cayenne pepper, 3 tbsp balsamic vinegar and 3 tbsp oil oil.

Put the tomatoes into a large bowl and coat them with this mixture. Arrange them in a single layer on the grids, cut side up and put them uncovered into the oven to cook for one to one and a half hours. Open the door every half hour to let out the steam. When they are cooked to outside of the tomato will be quite hard but there will still be quite a lot of moisture inside.

Oven dried tomatoes keep for a least a week in the fridge. To freeze them, put them onto a tray in a single layer and open freeze them. Once frozen pack them into boxes. You do not have to add any extra oil to them.

Red Bean, Avocado & Tomato Salad

You can use fresh or oven dried tomatoes to make this. The oven dried tomatoes give the salad a very intense flavour. If you do not have a preserved lemon, peel off 2 or 3 thin strips of rind from an unwaxed lemon. Dissolve 1 tsp salt in 5 tbsp of water and soak the lemon rind for about ½ hour. Drain it and then chop it finely.

SERVES 2 - 4

400g/14 oz can red beans
drained and rinsed
100g/3½oz feta cut into
5mm/¼ in dice
16 large oven dried tomatoes
1 small red onion finely chopped
2 large ripe avocados
Juice of 1 lemon

30g/1oz rocket or baby spinach
1 preserved lemon
2 tbsp toasted sunflower and pumpkin
seeds (optional)
30g/1oz ready made basil pesto

1 Remove the seeds from the preserved lemon and chop it finely. Cut the oven dried tomatoes in half.

2 Cut the avocados in half and remove the stones using a small spoon. Peel them and then chop them into 1cm/½ in dice. Sprinkle over 2 tablespoons of the lemon juice to prevent them turning brown. Mix the rest of the lemon juice with the pesto.

3 Put all the ingredients into a large bowl and gently mix them together.

Pickled Red Onions

These onions are a useful addition to salads and baked vegetables. They can be made in advance and kept in the fridge for several days. The marinade from them can be used as a dressing for salads. It is particularly good when it is mixed with pesto.

450g / 1 lb small red onions
90ml / 3 fl oz olive oil

90ml / 3 fl oz balsamic vinegar
Juice of a lemon

1 Peel the onions. If they are small, about the size of a large walnut, leave them whole, otherwise cut them in half or quarters.

2 Warm the oil and balsamic vinegar but do not let it boil.

3 Bring a pan or water to the boil. Add the onions, bring the water back to the boil and simmer the onions for 2 minutes. Drain and add them to the vinegar and oil. Add the lemon juice and optionally some zest of the lemon peeled in strips. Season with ground black pepper.

4 Leave the onions to marinade, turning every now and again. Leave for at least 3 hours before serving.

Pesto & Pickled Red Onion Salad

*This is one of those flexible salads that can be made with potatoes,
butter beans or cannellini beans and more or less any salad vegetables
that you have available. The Pickled red onions mixed with the pesto
and parmesan flakes make an interesting dressing.*

SERVES 4 - 6

6 pickled baby red onions -

12 small cooked salad potatoes

225g /8oz cooked French beans

6 small cooked artichoke hearts

6 spring onions shredded

30g/1oz basil pesto

Juice of half a lemon

3 tbsp fluid from the red onions

1 clove of crushed garlic (optional)

125g / 4oz baby plum tomatoes cut into
halves

18 stoned black olives

80g/3oz baby salad leaves or rocket

parmesan flakes

1 Cut the potatoes into halves and squeeze the lemon juice over
   them. Cook the French beans for 2 to 3 minutes until just al dente.
   Drain and refresh them in cold water.

2 To make the dressing, mix the pesto with the crushed garlic and
   the fluid from the pickled red onions.

3 Mix all the ingredients other than the salad leaves together and stir
   in the dressing. Add the salad leaves just before serving. Finish the
   salad with the parmesan flakes.

Salmon & Cauliflower Carpaccio

This is one of those meals that is quick to get onto the table as all of the vegetables can be prepared in advance and stored in the fridge. You will find the recipe for watercress pesto in the Herbs and Spices section.

SERVES 4

1 medium cauliflower

85g/3oz watercress

2 tbsp lemon juice

Small bunch of chives finely snipped

175g/6oz cooked, peeled prawns

175g/6 oz cooked salmon broken into bite size pieces

70g/2½oz watercress pesto

½ clove garlic crushed (optional)

For the Cauliflower Mayo

30g/1oz butter

150ml/5 fl oz milk

2 tsp grated horseradish

200g/7oz trimmings from the cauliflower

1   Quarter the cauliflower, then slice each quarter into 5mm/¼in pieces. Cut as many long slices as you can and break the rest into small thumb size florets. Reserves the trimmings for the cauliflower mayonnaise.

2   Bring a large pan of water to the boil and add the cauliflower slices. You will probably need to do this is two batches. Bring them back to the boil and cook for 2 minutes. Lift them out and put them into a bowl of cold water. When you have finished with the slices do the same with the florets.

3   To make the cauliflower mayonnaise, heat a medium size pan, add the butter and milk and 200g/7oz of the trimmings from the cauliflower. Bring to the boil - keep your eye on it in case it boils over. Reduce the heat to low and cook for 10 minutes until the cauliflower is tender.

4   Purée the cauliflower, milk and butter in a food processor or blend it with a hand blender. Leave it to cool and then add the horseradish and 1 tbsp lemon juice. Blend until it is smooth.

5   If you are using it, mix the crushed garlic into the watercress pesto.

6   To serve, wash and dry the prawns and mix them with the chives. Put the cauliflower and watercress into a large serving bowl, add the prawns, chives and pieces of salmon. Drizzle some of the cauliflower mayo over.

Serve the watercress pesto and the rest of the cauliflower mayonnaise in separate bowls.

Alfalfa, Avocado & Salmon Salad

SERVES 2

200g/7oz cooked salmon or trout with skin and bones removed
A large handful of alfalfa
A punnet of mustard cress
2 large ripe avocados

Small bunch of chives finely sliced
Juice of 1 lemon
1 tbsp Thai fish sauce
Baby gem lettuce to serve

1   Wash the alfalfa and mustard cress and spin them dry.

2   Flake the fish into bite size pieces and put it into a bowl with the mustard cress, alfalfa and chives. Mix the lemon juice and Thai fish sauce together in a jar.

3   When you are ready to serve the salad cut the avocados in half and remove the stone using a small spoon. Peel them and cut them into 1cm/½ in dice. Put them into the bowl with the other ingredients and pour on the lemon juice. Serve the salad on a bed of baby gem lettuce leaves.

Carrot Chicory & Rocket Salad

SERVES 4 - 6

Dressing

2tbsp olive oil

1 tbsp walnut oil

1tbsp cider or white wine vinegar

1 tbsp lemon juice

1 tsp clear honey

1 tsp finely grated lemon zest

3 medium size carrots

1 large head of chicory

60g/2oz rocket or watercress

1   Separate the leaves of chicory and cut them in half lengthways. Put them into a large bowl.

2   Peel and grate the carrot and add it to the chicory. Then add the rocket and mix everything together.

3   Put all of the ingredients for the dressing into a screw top jar and give them a good shake. Just before serving toss the salad in the dressing.

Cucumber Salad

This is a simple delicate salad that goes really well with cold salmon and trout. It can also be served with curries.

SERVES

½ telegraph cucumber

1 tsp finely chopped parsley or chervil

1 tsp Thai fish sauce

Juice and grated zest of ½ lime

50ml/2fl oz water

Peel the cucumber, cut it in half and remove the seeds. Slice it very thinly and mix it with the other ingredients.

French Bean, Roquefort & Nut Salad

You can use pecan nuts or walnuts and any type of blue cheese to make this. The Omega-3 oils in the nuts counters the inflammatory effect of the cheese.

SERVES 4

300g/10½oz fine French beans

150g/5½oz Roquefort or other blue cheese broken into small pieces

100g/3½oz pecan nuts or walnuts roughly chopped

1 large or 2 small baby gem lettuce

3 tbsp olive oil

1 tbsp Balsamic vinegar

1   Cook the French beans in boiling water for 3 minutes until they are just tender. Drain and rinse them in cold water.

2   Wash and dry the lettuce and cut it into pieces lengthways.

3   Put the olive oil and balsamic vinegar into a jar and give it a shake.

4   Mix the lettuce, French beans, walnuts together and sprinkle over the cheese. Cover and refrigerate.

5   Just before serving stir in a half of the dressing. Serve the rest of the dressing in a separate bowl.

Chinese Leaf, Pepper & Sweetcorn Salad

Chinese leaf is a valuable store cupboard ingredient as it is available all the year round and it keeps well. This is a bright, colourful salad that will keep for 2 days in a covered container in the fridge. Serve it on its own or with a dressing of your choice.

SERVES 4 - 6

1 large sweet Ramiro pepper

325g/11 ½oz can sweetcorn kernels

4 spring onions finely sliced

½ Chinese Leaf Cabbage

2 punnets of mustard cress

1   Remove the seeds from the red pepper and cut it into thin rings. Finely shred the Chinese Leaf.

2   Rinse and drain the sweetcorn kernels, put them into a large bowl and mix them with the mustard cress.

3   Stir in the red pepper and Chinese Leaf and the spring onions.

Potato, Dill Cucumber & Walnut Salad
A salad that goes well with fish and seafood.

SERVES 4

6 spring onions finely sliced

450g/1lb cooked waxy salad potatoes

150g/5½oz small pickled gherkins or dill cucumbers

4 tbsp fromage frais or natural unsweetened yoghurt

60g/2¼oz pecan nuts or walnuts coarsely chopped

Hand full of parsley, chervil or dill finely chopped

1   Either cut the cooked potatoes into ½ cm/¼ in slices or cut them into 1cm/½ in dice. Slice the gherkins into thin rounds.

2   Put the yoghurt into a large bowl and add the parsley, chervil or dill, the chopped nuts and the spring onions.

3   Add the potatoes and the sliced gherkins. Give everything a good stir and pile it onto a serving plate.

Potato & Cucumber Salsa

This salsa can be served with any type of shellfish as well as salmon and trout. It will keep in the fridge for 2 days.

SERVES 4

24 small cooked new potatoes
1 large telegraph cucumber, peeled,
cut in half lengthways and de-seeded
8 spring onions finely chopped
1 finely chopped green chilli
1 - 2 cloves of garlic crushed
3 tbsp capers drained and roughly
chopped

1 tbsp finely chopped fresh dill
1 tbsp chopped flat leaf parsley
or chervil
Finely grated zest of 2 limes
Juice of 2 limes
2 tbsp olive oil
Sprigs of fresh dill or parsley to garnish.

1   Cut the potatoes and cucumber into small 5mm/¼ in dice and put them into a large bowl.

2   Add the spring onions, chilli, garlic, capers, dill, parsley and lime zest and give everything a good stir.

3   Put the lime juice and olive oil into a small jar, put on the lid and give it a good shake. Mix this into the potato and cucumber mixture. Chill before serving.

Beetroot, French Bean & Haloumi Salad

If you can find them, use cooked baby beetroot. Failing that cut larger pre cooked beetroot into bite size segments.

SERVES 2

275/10oz cooked beetroot

125g/4 ½oz haloumi cut into
5mm/¼ in slices

2 tbsp olive oil

1 - 2 tsp cumin seeds lightly toasted

150g/6oz fine French beans topped
and tailed

4 tbsp balsamic vinegar

Dash of Tabasco (optional)

Crushed black pepper

1   Bring a pan of water to the boil, add the French beans. Bring them to the boil and cook for 3 minutes until they are just tender. Drain, refresh them in cold water and drain again.

2   Pre heat the grill to high. If the beetroot are small leave them whole, other wise cut them into segments. Put them onto a greased baking tray with the haloumi. Brush the beetroot and haloumi with 1 tbsp of the oil and grill for 4 or 5 minutes. Keep an eye it as the haloumi can burn quite easily.

3   Mix the remaining oil, Tabasco and balsamic vinegar together in a large bowl. Add the green beans, beetroot and haloumi, mix well and sprinkle on the toasted cumin seeds.

Serve straight away.

Sweet Potato, Avocado & Tofu

To make this recipe you need the orange variety of sweet potato. The avocados need to be perfectly ripe. The polenta dusting freezes well so it is worth making a batch for the freezer.

SERVES 4

200g/6½oz firm tofu or Tempeh cut into finger size pieces about 5cm/2 in long
2 large sweet potatoes weighing 400g/12oz
200g/6½ oz baby plum tomatoes
2 large avocados or 3 medium ones
50g/1½oz rocket or baby spinach

For the polenta dusting
100g/3½oz medium polenta
½ clove garlic crushed (optional)
2 large handfuls of fresh basil or coriander
1 egg beaten
Mixed salad leaves to serve

For the dressing:
2 tbsp olive oil
1 tbsp wholegrain mustard
1 tbsp balsamic vinegar
2 tbsp lemon or lime juice

1   Pre heat the oven to 180°C/ 350°F/Gas 4

2   To make the polenta dusting, wash and dry the basil or coriander. Put it into a blender with the polenta and, if you are using it the garlic, and whiz until the coriander is amalgamated with the polenta. The polenta will turn pale green.

3   Peel and slice the sweet potatoes into 1cm/½ in slices. Put them onto a baking tray lined with non stick foil and brush them lightly with oil. Bake them for about 15 minutes until they are tender. Take them out and leave them to cool. Leave the oven on.

4   Heat some olive oil in an oven proof non stick pan on a moderate heat. Dip the tofu into the beaten egg and then coat it with the polenta. Put the tofu into the pan and cook it over a medium heat.

After one side has set and turned golden turn the polenta over and put the pan into oven. Roast the tofu for 10 minutes.

5   To make the dressing put the balsamic vinegar, grain mustard, lemon or lime juice and olive oil into a jar. Put on the lid and give it a good shake.

6   Cut the avocados in half, take out the stones using a small spoon and cut them into chunks. Mix them with the dressing straight away to prevent them from turning brown. Add the tomatoes, cut in half, and the cooked sweet potato. Gently stir in the cooked tofu.

Serve with salad leaves or baby spinach.

Goats Cheese & Walnut Salad

A simple salad that takes only minutes to prepare. Goats cheese, walnuts or pecan nuts and red beans go together really well. If you don't like goats cheese use Camembert or Brie instead.

SERVES 4

250g/9oz Chevre log cut into16 pieces

16 slices from a small baguette cut ½ cm/¼ in thick

70g/2½oz packet of mixed baby salad leaves

400g/14 oz can red beans drained and rinsed

85g/3oz walnuts or pecan nuts roughly chopped

Small bunch chives cut into 2cm/1 in pieces

For the dressing:

1 tbsp walnut oil

1 tbsp lemon juice

½ tsp chilli paste or Sambol Oelek

1   Set the grill onto high and toast the slices of baguette on one side.

2   Put the salad leaves into a large bowl with the red beans and the walnuts. Mix the walnut oil, chilli and lemon juice together and mix it into the salad and beans. Divide the salad between 4 plates.

3   Put the slices of Chevre onto the un-toasted side of the baguette and grill it until it turns a light golden brown. Keep an eye on it as it burns very easily.

4   Arrange 4 pieces of the grilled Chevre log on top of the salad and serve immediately.

Pumpkin, French Bean & Feta Salad

You can use pumpkin, butternut squash or orange sweet potatoes to make this salad. Use walnut oil or olive oil if you do not have any pumpkin oil.

SERVES 4

1¼Kg/2lb 13oz pumpkin peeled
and cut into chunks or wedges
200g/7oz fine French beans
200g/7oz crumbled feta
3 tbsp toasted pumpkin seeds

For the dressing:
2 tbsp pumpkin seed oil
Finely grated zest and juice of a lemon
½ tsp smoked garlic granules (optional)

Pre heat the oven to 200°C/400°F/Gas 5.

1   Put the pumpkin onto a tray lined with non stick foil and bake for 20 minutes until tender.

2   Boil the French beans for 3 – 4 minutes until they are just tender, drain and refresh them in cold water.

3   Make the dressing by putting all of the ingredients into a jar and giving them a good shake.

4   Put the pumpkin and French beans into a large bowl and stir in the dressing.

5   Divide the pumpkin and French beans between 4 plates, scatter with the toasted pumpkin seeds and the crumbled feta. Serve immediately.

Roasted Tomato, Feta & Lentil Salad

Puy lentils are a useful store cupboard ingredient as they do not need to be soaked before they are cooked.

SERVES 4

100g/3½oz Puy lentils	200g/7oz feta OR 4 hard boiled eggs cut
300ml/10 fl oz (½pt) water	into quarters
12 medium size tomatoes cut in half	2 punnets of mustard cress
1 tbsp balsamic vinegar	large handful of basil leaves
1 tsp sea salt flakes	Juice ½ lemon
6 spring onions sliced	

Pre heat the oven to 200ºC/ 400ºF/Gas 5

1   Wash and drain the lentils and put them into a saucepan with the water. Bring them to the boil, cover and reduce the heat to low. Simmer them for 40 to 45 minutes until they are tender. Drain off any liquid that is left.

2   Put the tomatoes cut side up onto a baking tray lined with non stick foil. Sprinkle over the salt and drizzle over the balsamic vinegar. Roast the tomatoes for 30 minutes.

3   Put the lentils into a large bowl and stir in the lemon juice. Add the tomatoes, sliced spring onions and the mustard cress or watercress.

4   Divide between 4 plates and scatter over the crumbled feta or boiled egg

HERBS, SPICES, NUTS & SEEDS

Herbs and spices have been around for thousands of years and they form a staple part of the diet of many countries. Indian, Asian and North African food all gain their characteristic flavours from herbs and spices.

As well as adding flavour to your food, herbs and spices also contain large amounts of flavonoids, anthocyanins and phytonutrients. These have powerful antioxidant, anti-inflammatory and medicinal properties. Chilli peppers, garlic, ginger, turmeric, rosemary, bay leaves, cumin, coriander, dill, fennel, oregano, sage and thyme are all great and their use in cooking as well as in medicine goes back a long way. Just half a teaspoon of dried garlic, chilli or ginger can transform an inflammatory food into an anti-inflammatory one.

Parsley and chervil have attracted a lot of attention recently as they are both very rich sources of flavonoids, Vitamin C and the beta carotene from which Vitamin A is made. They also contain a very powerful oil called Myristicin which activates an enzyme that works with one of our body's antioxidants to neutralise free radicals. Interestingly, in the middle ages, parsley and chervil were used by the monks as a cure for gout.

Nuts and seeds are complex foods that contain many different nutrients, some of which are known to reduce chronic and systemic inflammation. Most are loaded with Essential Fatty Acids that are in a 'natural' ratio and they bring with them their own supply of antioxidants and vitamins that stop the oil inside the nuts from oxidising. Brazil nuts, walnuts, pecan nuts, almonds, hazelnuts, pumpkin seeds, sesame seeds, flax seeds, in fact all nuts and seeds are good and they are great for snacking on. Healthy they may be but all nuts are high in calories so eat them in moderation.

Isn't the Omega-6 EFA one of the not so good oils? Well nuts and seeds are not just tiny packets of Omega-3 and Omega-6. They are a long way from the heat processed polyunsaturated vegetable oils. As nuts and seeds are something a tree or plant grows from they are a pretty complete source of nutrition; fats, carbohydrates, and protein plus vitamins like vitamin E, minerals and antioxidants that all work together to protect the fats from becoming oxidised. When we strip the oil from the seed it doesn't have any of these things to protect it and this is when the trouble starts. A hand full of nuts bares no resemblance to a spoonful of vegetable oil.

Only buy natural uncooked nuts and seeds. Commercially roasted nuts and seeds usually contain a lot of additives and you have no control over how long they have been roasted for or the temperature they have been roasted at. Polyunsaturated vegetable oils are also often added as part of the roasting process. You can soak nuts overnight to make them plump and succulent like fresh ones or roast them lightly. If you cook them for too long or at too high a temperature the oils in them oxidise and the antioxidants they contain are reduced.

Making Pesto

Pestos are a really good way of using herbs as they enable you to eat the herbs raw and this preserves not only their flavour but also their nutritional value. Adding lemon or lime juice to the pesto preserves its colour by slowing down the rate at which it oxidises.

You can use pesto on its own, stirred into yoghurt to make dips and added to vegetables and grains. Mixed with toasted oatmeal or Panko (Japanese) breadcrumbs and optionally with a little grated parmesan or pecorino they make a wonderful crumb topping for fish and vegetables. Just about any herb can be made into pesto. Vegetables like beetroot and semi dried dried tomatoes can also be used. Black and green olives can be processed in exactly the same way to make tapenade.

Making pesto is a little time consuming and it is certainly not something you want to do every day. However, the good news is that pesto freezes well and freezing does not destroy any of the pesto's nutritional value. If you are going to make some pesto it is worthwhile making a large batch and freezing it in small portions. Just remember to leave out the garlic as after a few weeks in the freezer it will start to develop a slight musty flavour. You can always add garlic when you thaw the pesto out.

How do you freeze pesto? All you need to do is open freeze large spoon fulls on a tray lined with cling film and when the pesto is frozen use some foil to wrap it up into individual parcels. It is also worthwhile investing in some small silicon muffin tins and using these to hold the pesto while it is being frozen.

Basil Pesto

The 'pesto' we all think of as pesto. Like coriander pesto, this is so useful it is worth making it in large quantities. Most recipes for basil pesto use pine nuts but any type of nut will do.

300g/10½oz basil
100g/3½oz raw cashew nuts
30g/1oz lightly toasted sunflower seeds

10 tbsp olive oil
85g/3oz finely grated parmesan
Crushed garlic to taste

1   Wash and dry the basil and remove any coarse stems.

2   Put the cashew nuts and sunflower seeds into a food processor and grind them.

3   Add the basil to the food processor. You will need to do this in stages as there will be too much basil to go in in one go. When the basil has reduced in volume add the other ingredients and blend well.

Olive & Almond Spread

This is a rich and concentrated spread that is in between a pesto and a tapenade. In terms of flavour a little goes a long way.

100g/3½oz pitted black olives
100g/3½oz ground almonds
1 tbsp capers
1 tbsp olive oil

Crushed garlic (optional)
1 tsp Sambol Oelek

Put everything into a blender and blend into a purée. Add a little water if the mixture looks too dry.

Gremolata

This is an adaptation of the classical Italian gremolata which is a
mixture of very finely chopped parsley and lemon juice. You can use
any type of nut but make sure you use flat leaf parsley and not curled
parsley as it has a much better flavour.

250g/9 oz flat leaf parsley	Finely grated zest of a lemon
50g/1¾oz walnuts or pecan nuts	Juice of a lemon
3 tbsp olive oil	Garlic to taste
1 tbsp finely grated parmesan	Salt to taste

Remove any coarse stems from the parsley and then wash and drain
it. If necessary dry it in some kitchen paper. Roughly chop it. Grind the
walnuts to a fairly fine powder in a food processor. Add all the other
ingredients and blend until everything is well mixed into a thick
purée.

Rocket Pesto

100g/3½oz rocket	1 tbsp white wine vinegar
50g/1¾oz grated parmesan	50g/1¾oz ground almonds
½ tsp grain mustard	4 tbsp olive oil
1 tsp Sambol Oelek or chilli paste	Crushed garlic to taste
Juice ½ lemon	

Wash and dry the rocket and remove any tough leaves. Put everything
into a food processor and blend until fully mixed.

Coriander Pesto

Having coriander pesto in the freezer is really useful, especially when you are making curries.

175g/6oz coriander leaves and stems	Finely grated zest of a lime
3 tbsp whole almonds with their skins	Juice of a lime
4 tbsp olive oil	1 tsp finely chopped chilli OR 1 tsp Sambol
Salt to taste	Oelek

1 Wash and dry the coriander. Grind the almonds to a fine powder in a blender or food processor.

2 Roughly chop the coriander and add it with the other ingredients to the almonds in the food processor and blend until fully mixed.

Watercress Pesto

This goes really well with salmon and trout.

100g/3½oz watercress including stalks	2 small spring onions – white only
4 tbsp olive oil	1 tbsp ground almonds
1 tsp balsamic vinegar	

Wash and dry the watercress. Put everything into a blender and whiz it into a paste

Beetroot Pesto

Beetroot pesto makes a colourful, tasty dip for vegetables and it goes really well with salmon, trout and herring. You can also stir it into quinoa, bulgar wheat and pasta.

250g/9oz packet of cooked beetroot roughly chopped
55g/2oz raw cashew nuts
Finely grated zest and juice of a lime
70g/2½oz finely grated parmesan

2 tbsp chopped parsley
3 heaped tsp grated horseradish
3 tbsp olive oil
Salt to taste
Crushed garlic to taste

Grind the cashew nuts in a food processor.

Add all the other ingredients and blitz until everything is well mixed into to a paste. Omit the garlic if you are making the pesto for the freezer.

Tapenade

You can make tapenade with either black or green olives. If you are using black olives try to obtain the dry salted ones from Turkey or Morocco as they have a much finer flavour and they are less likely to have been dyed.

85g/3oz pitted black olives
4 anchovy fillets OR 2 tsp anchovy paste
35g/1¼oz capers

2 cloves garlic crushed or more or less to taste
4 tbsp olive oil
½ finely chopped red chilli (optional)

Put everything into a blender or food processor and blitz until you have a smooth but grainy paste.

Oven Roasted Tomato Pesto
You can make this with oven dried tomatoes or sun dried tomatoes.

16 oven roasted tomato halves
30g/1oz finely grated parmesan
1 tbsp crushed garlic
1 tbsp olive oil

4 – 5 large basil leaves
pinch of cayenne pepper or dash of red
Tabasco

Put everything into a blender and mix well.

Yellow Thai Curry Paste
If you do not have any lemon grass use the finely grated zest of a lemon instead.

6 orange or yellow chillies
1 stalk of lemon grass
4 shallots
4 cloves of garlic sliced
1 tbsp grated ginger
1 tbsp brown sugar

1 tsp coriander seeds
1 tsp mustard powder
½ tsp turmeric
1 tsp salt
½ tsp ground cinnamon
2 tbsp olive oil

Put all the ingredients into a blender or pestle and mortar and blend thoroughly. Store in a covered container in the fridge.

Spicy North African Relish

This a combination of Chermoula and Harrisa, a taste of North Africa that goes really well with fish and vegetables. It is especially good with tortillas and frittatas. You can adjust the amount of chilli or Sambol Oelek to suit your taste. Remember to leave out the garlic if you are freezing it.

85g/3oz coriander

85g/3oz flat leaf parsley

1 large Ramiro pepper weighing about

150g/5½oz

2 tbsp ground cumin

1 tsp ground coriander

1 tsp dried mint

1 tbsp sweet paprika

1 small red chilli OR 2 tsp Sambol Oelek

2 tbsp olive oil

Finely grated zest of a lemon

Juice of a lemon

Crushed garlic to taste

1   Cut the Ramiro pepper in half lengthways and remove the seeds. Put it on a microwave plate, cover and microwave of full power for 4 minutes.

2   De seed and roughly chop the chilli if you are using it.

3   Roughly chop the Ramiro pepper and put it into a food processor or blender with the other ingredients. Blend until you have a smooth paste. If the paste looks a bit too thick add some more olive oil.

How To Make Tamarind Pulp

Tamarind has a distinctive tart, sour flavour. It is always available in Asian supermarkets as it is widely used in Asian food. You can also buy it on the Internet. If you are unable to obtain tamarind you can use lemon or lime juice instead.

With the exception of fresh tamarind which you will only find in Asian food stores, there are two ways you can buy tamarind. One is a block of compressed tamarind fruit that looks a bit like a block of dried dates. The other is a small tub of tamarind concentrate. The tamarind concentrate is the easiest to use but the compressed tamarind has a much better flavour.

All you need to do to use the tamarind concentrate is to dissolve a tablespoon in 3 tablespoons of boiling water.

Compressed Tamarind is usually sold in blocks of 450g. To make tamarind pulp, tear up the block into small pieces and place them in a stainless steel or non metallic bowl. Cover with 1Lt/1¾ pt/35 fl oz very hot water and set it aside overnight or for at least 5 hours to soak.

Pour the soaked tamarind into a sieve over a stainless steel or non metallic bowl. Using a wooden spoon push as much pulp as possible through the sieve. Don't forget to collect all the thick, strained paste that clings to the underneath of the sieve and stir this in. A 450g block of tamarind should yield about 350ml/12 fl oz of pulp.

Spoon the pulp into ice cube trays or small muffin cases in approximately 2 tbsp amounts and freeze. Once frozen the pulp can be put into a bag or box and stored for up to a year.

Nuts & Seeds

Nuts and seeds form an important part of an anti inflammatory diet as they are all anti inflammatory and packed full of anti oxidants and healthy micro nutrients. As with all things nuts and seeds are not created equal and some are more anti inflammatory than others. Interestingly Brazil nuts are almost off the scale when it comes to their anti inflammatory properties. The only thing to remember is that all nuts and seeds contain a lot of calories, so even thought they are healthy consume them in moderation.

Only buy natural nuts and seeds. When nuts and seeds are roasted and toasted commercially oils and additives are often added.

Toasting & Roasting Nuts & Seeds

Lightly toasting and roasting nuts and seeds brings out their natural flavours and freshens them up if they have become a bit stale. You can toast nuts and seeds in the oven, in the microwave and on the hob. Large nuts like whole almonds and hazelnuts are better if they are lightly roasted in the oven.

To toast them in the oven heat the oven to 180°C/ 350°F/Gas 4. Put the nuts and seeds in a single layer on a baking tray and cook them for precisely 8 minutes. I think it was Delia Smith who first said "precisely 8 minutes" and she is absolutely right. Cook them for any longer and they will burn.

To toast nuts and seeds in a microwave, spread them out on a large plate and cook them uncovered on HIGH for 4 – 5 minutes until they are lightly browned.

If you are toasting hazelnuts roll them in a damp cloth or some damp kitchen paper after you have toasted them to rub off the loose brown skin.

To toast nuts and seeds in a saucepan, put the saucepan over a medium heat. Keep stirring them and don't let them get too brown. Remember, when you take them off the heat they will carry on cooking for a bit.

Nut Butters

Nut butters are useful things to have around and they are surprisingly easy to make, provided of course that you have a food processor or blender. The benefit of making them yourself is that you are in control of how much sugar, if any, they contain and also how long they have been roasted for and the type of oil that is used.

If you look on the internet you will find a lot of recipes for nut butters. Many of these recipes soak the nuts and then dry them before making the nut butter. The reasoning behind this is that by soaking the nuts and discarding the soaking water you remove the phytic acid that they contain. This is a natural 'anti-nutrient' that adversely affects the way our bodies absorb some trace elements and minerals. The theory is that by removing the phytic acid you also make the nut butter easier to digest. The only problem with this is that the soaking process also removes the polyphenols or tannins that the nuts' contain as well as many of the other micro nutrients that your body needs.

You can use any type of nut or seed to make nut butter. Because of the large amount of oil they contain Brazil nuts make really good nut butter, especially when combined with other nuts. You can use the nuts in their natural state and you can also lightly roast or toast them, either in the oven, on the hob or under the grill to bring out their flavour. Whether you sweeten the nut butter is purely a matter of taste. If you do sweeten them honey, natural Maple syrup or raw cane sugar are probably the best choices, but remember that are still 'sugar'. If you want to flavour them you can add any spice that you like, ground cinnamon, ground nutmeg or ground ginger are all good. Add these at the end of the processing.

Nut butters will keep for three to four weeks in the fridge but they also freeze well and once frozen can be kept for up to 6 months. So the best advice is to make a large batch and then freeze the nut butter in small amounts. Remember, nut butters may be healthy but they are VERY high in calories.

Almond Butter

Use whole as opposed to blanched almonds to make this. If you want to roast the almonds to bring out their flavour cook them for 8 minutes at 180°C/ 350°F/Gas 4. Leave them until they are completely cold before processing them.

Pulse 200g/7oz of almonds in a food processor or blender until you have quite a fine powder. The powder will work its way up the sides of the food processor so every now and then take off the lid and scrape it back down.

Keep processing. The nuts will begin to form a stiff lumpy mass.

Carry on processing until the almonds begin to release their oil and form a smooth paste. This will take between 5 to10 minutes or may be even longer, and the paste will become slightly warm. At this stage you can add a tablespoon or two of oil, almond oil, coconut oil, olive oil or what ever you have available and process until you have a thick creamy paste. Whatever you do don't add any water. If you do you will end up with an unpleasant slurry. You can add 50g/1¾oz of sunflower, sesame of pumpkin seeds toward the end of the processing time if you want the butter to have a crunchy texture. Store in a sealed jar in the fridge or freeze in small quantities.

Nut Free Butter

You can make nut free butters with sunflower seeds, pumpkin seeds and sesame seeds. Lightly toast the seeds first as this brings out their flavour. If you want to make a 'sweet' butter to 200g/7oz lightly toasted sunflower seeds add 1 tsp ground nutmeg, 1 tsp ground cinnamon, ½ tsp ground ginger and 1 tbsp dark unrefined muscavado sugar or Maple syrup at the end.

Hazelnut & Chocolate Spread

A home made version of hazelnut and chocolate spread and making it is easier than you think. A recipe for hazelnut and chocolate parfait that uses this recipe is included in the desserts section.

200g/7oz hazelnuts
3 tbsp cocoa powder
3 heaped tbsp dark unrefined muscavado sugar

50g/1¾oz butter
1 tsp vanilla extract
2 tbsp water + 6 tbsp water

Pre heat the oven to 180°C/ 350°F/Gas 4

1   Put the hazelnuts onto a baking tray and roast them for precisely 8 minutes. This will bring out their flavour.

2   Take them out of the oven, put them into a damp tea towel and rub them. Most of the skins will come off, don't worry about any that are left on.

3   Process the hazelnuts as described above until they release their oil and form a smooth paste. This will take between 5 and 10 minutes.

4   Put 2 tbsp water, the butter, the cocoa powder and the sugar into a small saucepan and gently heat it until the butter is melted. Keep stirring it over a low heat and cook it for 3 – 4 minutes. This will take the raw taste out of the cocoa.

5   Stir in 1 tsp vanilla extract and leave the mixture to cool slightly.

6   Pour the chocolate mixture into the hazelnuts and process. Slowly add 6 tbsp cold water, 1 tbsp at a time until you have a smooth slightly runny paste.

You can keep the hazelnut and chocolate spread in a covered container in the fridge or freeze it in small quantities.

Gomasio

Gomasio or gomashio is a seasoning blend that is sprinkled on simple rice dishes in Japan. It tastes really good sprinkled on stir fries, cooked vegetables and salads. It is very simple to make as the only ingredients are sesame seeds and salt. You can use white, black or brown sesame seeds. For 15 teaspoons of sesame seeds you will need 1 teaspoon of coarse sea salt crystals.

Heat a saucepan over a medium heat and put in the salt. Stir it around for a minute to dry it. Take it out of the saucepan and put it to one side

Lightly toast the sesame seeds in the saucepan for 1 – 2 minutes, just long enough to bring out the flavour and colour them slightly. When they are ready they will start to pop and smell 'nutty'.

When the sesame seeds are cold put them into a blender or pestle and mortar and grind them until about half of the seeds have been crushed. Add the sea salt crystals and give them a quick whiz to mix everything together and break down the crystals

Store in an airtight container in the fridge as the gomasio oxidises and goes rancid very quickly after it is made.

Za-atar

A mixture of herbs and spices that you can sprinkle on salads and vegetables. Recipes are handed down in families and the herbs, spices and proportions in which they are used all vary. You can make the Za-atar in larger amounts than in the following recipe and store it in an airtight container for several weeks.

2 tsp dried oregano

1 tsp sumac

1 tsp toasted sesame seeds

1 tsp ground cumin

Pinch chilli flakes

Pinch sea salt flakes

Put everything into a blender or grinder and give it a quick blitz. You do not need to make it into a fine powder. Store it in an airtight container.

Dukkah

A mixture of nuts, herbs and spices that you can sprinkle onto salads and vegetables.

70g/2½oz toasted hazelnuts

70g/2½oz toasted sesame seeds

2 tbsp cumin seeds

2 tbsp coriander seeds

1 tbsp sweet paprika

1 tbsp onion seeds

2 tbsp dessicated coconut

Lightly toast the cumin, onion and coriander seeds in a saucepan, just long enough to bring out the flavour. Do the same with the coconut. When everything is cold put it into a blender with the other ingredients and blend until you have a coarse powder. Store in an airtight container.

PATES, DIPS & SAUCES

Eat them on their own, with salad and vegetables, serve them as starters or eat them with crudités.

Guacamole

They say that an authentic Guacamole contains only avocado, fresh coriander, tomato and fresh chillies. If you add anything else to it it becomes an avocado dip.

You can use this recipe as a dip by adding some natural unsweetened yoghurt and serve it with raw vegetables and pieces of Socca and you can use it as a sauce with cold fish and bean dishes and with Mexican burgers. When serving it with beans it works really well with red beans.

Use really ripe avocados for the best results. You can alter the proportions of the various ingredients to suit your taste.

SERVES

2 to 3 fresh chillies finely chopped
OR 2 tsp Sambol Oelek
2 medium tomatoes finely chopped
1 tbsp finely chopped onion
1 clove garlic crushed

2 tbsp chopped fresh coriander
2 large or 3 medium ripe avocados
Lemon or lime juice to taste

1   Peel and mash the avocado and mix it with the other ingredients.

2   Add 1 or 2 tablespoons of lemon juice and mix well. Leave the stone in the guacamole until you are ready to eat it as for some reason this slows down the oxidation process.

3   Do not refrigerate. If you do the guacamole will go brown.

Baba Ganoush - Aubergine Pâté

This is a traditional Middle Eastern dish that is usually made with aubergines that have been 'charred' over an open flame. This gives the dish its characteristic smokey flavour. This is recipe is quicker and easier to make as it uses aubergine that is cooked in the microwave. Although it is not authentic, adding some smoked paprika and smoked garlic adds a slightly exotic smokey flavour. This pâté can be kept in the fridge for 2 to 3 days. It also freezes well.

1 large aubergine	2 tbsp Tahini
2 tbsp olive oil	ground black pepper
Juice of a lime juice of ½ a lemon	1 tbsp finely chopped coriander
½ tsp smoked paprika	Salt and pepper to taste
1 tsp smoked garlic	

1 Slice the aubergine into 5mm ¼ inch rounds and put them into a microwave bowl. Cover and cook on full power for 5 minutes. Give them a stir and cook them for another 3 minutes.

2 Leave the aubergine to cool a little with the cover on.

3 Add the smoked garlic and smoked paprika, the Tahini, lemon juice, black pepper and olive oil and blend until you have a smooth fluffy purée.. Stir in the chopped coriander.

4 If you want to make this into a creamy type of dip mix in one or two tablespoons of unsweetened yoghurt.

Cannellini Bean Pate

You can use cannellini beans or butter beans to make this. Serve the pate with crudités, with burgers and with salads made from quinoa, bulgar wheat and couscous.

SERVES 2 - 4

400g 14oz can of cannellini beans

3 tbsp natural unsweetened yoghurt
OR soft cheese like ricotta

Juice of a lemon

½ tsp chilli paste, Sambol Oelek or some finely chopped red chilli

1 clove crushed garlic

10 oven dried tomatoes or sun blushed tomatoes

12 stoned salted black olives

8 basil leaves

1   Drain and rinse the cannellini beans and place them with the lemon juice, yoghurt or soft cheese, chilli and crushed garlic in a deep bowl. Whiz them with a blender until they are a smooth purée

2   Chop the oven dried tomatoes and black olives and shred the basil leaves. Mix the olives, basil and tomatoes with the bean purée. Cover and chill until needed.

Smoked Mackerel Pâté

This takes just minutes to make. It can be stored in the fridge for a day or two and it can be frozen for up to three months. The following recipe is really a guideline as you can vary the ingredients to suit yourself.

SERVES 3 - 4

200g/7oz packet of hot smoked mackerel.

Juice of a lemon

2 heaped tsp grated horseradish - or more to taste

¼ - ½ tsp crushed black pepper

1 - 2 tbsp unsweetened natural yoghurt

1   Begin by taking the skin off of the smoked mackerel and removing any bones.

2   Break up the fillets and put them into a bowl with the horseradish, lemon juice crushed black pepper and yoghurt. Use a hand blender to whiz everything together. Taste the pâté and optionally add more lemon juice, horseradish or yoghurt.

3   You can serve this pâté on its own, as a starter with a beetroot and cucumber salad, as part of a mezze or thinned down with some more yoghurt as a dip with crudités.

Hummus

An easy to prepare dip that is basically a purée of chick peas (Garbanzo beans), a paste made from sesame seeds called Tahini and lemon juice. The Tahini is an essential ingredient for authentic hummus but even without the Tahini you can make some interesting dips.

SERVES 2 - 4

400g can of chick peas that have been drained and rinsed

½ -1 clove crushed garlic

1 – 2 tbsp Tahini paste

2 - 3 tbsp lemon juice

Salt and black pepper to taste

Cold water

1 tsp sweet paprika

1 tsp lightly toasted cumin seeds (optional)

1   Put the chickpeas, garlic, Tahini, lemon juice and 2 tablespoons of cold water into a bowl and whiz it with a hand blender until it has a smooth, creamy consistency. Gradually add some more cold water if the hummus is too thick.

2   Season to taste with salt and ground black pepper and transfer to a serving dish. Cover and chill in the fridge.

3   Just before serving drizzle over some olive oil, a sprinkling of paprika and/or some lightly toasted cumin seeds.

Variations:

- Cut a preserved lemon in half and remove the seeds and most of the flesh. Finely chop the skin and add this to the hummus

- Make the hummus as above but omit the Tahini paste, the garlic and the yoghurt. Roast a red pepper for 15 minutes in a hot oven. Put it onto a plate and cover it with cling film. When it is cool enough to handle peel off the skin, break it into pieces and blend it, together with any juices that have seeped out, into the hummus

Miso, Tofu & Tahini Dip

Silken tofu can be made into dips and it is a very useful ingredient for people who are unable to eat dairy products. This is an interesting dip that can be served on its own, with crudités or used as a dressing for vegetables and noodles. It freezes well but leave out the garlic if you are going to freeze it and add it later.

350g/12oz silken tofu
2 cloves garlic crushed
2 tbsp white miso
8 tbsp Tahini
Juice of 1 lemon OR 2 limes

3 tbsp light soy sauce
Crushed black pepper to taste
4 tbsp finely sliced chives

Put everything together in a bowl and blend with a hand blender until you have a smooth paste. Stir in half of the chives, put the dip into a serving bowl and sprinkle the remaining chives on top.

Uppingham Pâté

This is a very old recipe for using up Blue Stilton cheese that has become a little 'tired'. Mature Blue Stilton makes the best Uppingham pâté but you can use any type of blue cheese. Served on its own this is quite an inflammatory dish but serving it with baby beetroot and some salad leaves or as a dip with carrot, celery and pepper crudités transforms it. The pâté can be kept in the fridge for 4 to 5 days. It can also be frozen for 1 to 2 months.

SERVES

700ml/25 fl oz/1¼pt milk

1 large onion roughly chopped

1 large carrot peeled and roughly chopped

2 stalks celery chopped

1 tsp dried mixed herbs

85g/3oz butter

85g/3oz flour

2 tbsp lemon juice

1 - 2 cloves garlic crushed

15 stoned green olives finely chopped

½ tsp salt

½ tsp black pepper

¼ – ½ tsp cayenne pepper

350g/12oz Stilton cheese rind removed and crumbled

1   Put the milk into a saucepan and add the onion, carrot, celery and mixed herbs. Bring to the boil, reduce the heat and simmer uncovered for 20 minutes.

2   Remove from the heat and leave it to cool a little. Strain the milk through a sieve into a large bowl, pressing with a wooden spoon to extract as much juice as possible from the vegetables. Discard the contents of the sieve and set the milk to one side.

3   Melt the butter in a saucepan over a medium heat. Whisk in the flour and cook for 2 minutes stirring constantly. Slowly whisk in the milk and cook until the sauce is thick and smooth. Turn the heat to very low and let the sauce cook for 5 minutes. Set the sauce aside to cool.

4   When the sauce is cool add the cheese, lemon juice, crushed garlic, salt pepper and cayenne. Use a hand blender to blend it until it is smooth, then stir in the chopped olives. Cover with cling film and chill for at least an hour before serving.

Simple Tahini Sauce or Dip

This is simply a mixture of sesame paste (Tahini) that is mixed in varying proportions to form a sauce or dip. You can mix the Tahini with:-

- *lemon juice and water,*

- *yoghurt and lemon juice or*

- *a mixture of lemon juice, yoghurt and water.*

The addition of crushed garlic is optional. Once made the Tahini will keep in the fridge for several days.

Caper & Coriander Vinaigrette

Serve this sauce warm or cold with fish or vegetables. Use coriander pesto from the freezer if you do not have any fresh coriander.

2 heaped tbsp finely chopped coriander	1 tsp wholegrain mustard
1 heaped tbsp capers roughly chopped	2 tbsp olive oil
½ clove garlic crushed	1 tbsp liquid from the capers
1 spring onion finely sliced	Salt and pepper to taste

Heat the oil in a small pan and lightly sauté the garlic and onion for 2 minutes. Add the rest of the ingredients and heat through.

Cucumber & Yoghurt Salad

This is a very simple salad type dip that is made from grated cucumber and yoghurt. This basic combination of ingredients is found all over the world. In Greece it is flavoured with garlic and dill and called Tzatziki and in India it is flavoured with mint and called Raita.

SERVES

1 large telegraph cucumber or 300g/11oz Lebanese cucumbers

½ tsp salt

1 - 2 cloves crushed garlic

1 tsp dried dill or more to taste

300ml/10 fl oz thick natural unsweetened yoghurt

1   The secret of making this and any other type of cucumber salad is to remove as much water as possible from the cucumber. In order to do this you will need an clean tea towel or some muslin.

2   Place the tea towel or muslin on a deep plate and coarsely grate the cucumber onto it. Gather up the tea towel and squeeze out as much of the fluid from the cucumber as you can. You will be amazed how much comes out.

3   Put the cucumber into a bowl and add ½ teaspoon of salt, a clove of crushed garlic and the dried dill. Give it a good stir and then add about two thirds of the yoghurt. Stir it round and if the mixture looks too thick add the rest of the yoghurt. How much you need to add depends on how much fluid was in the cucumber in the first place and how much you have managed to squeeze out. Add more garlic to taste.

Nut Butter & Coconut Cream Sauce

Using nut butters that you have ready made and then stored in the freezer saves a considerable amount of time. This is a sauce that can transform a terrine or simple plate of cooked vegetables into a substantial meal.

3 tbsp almond or cashew nut butter
50g/2 oz creamed coconut roughly chopped
200ml/7 fl oz boiling water

100g/4 oz silken tofu
1 tsp ground cumin
salt and pepper

1   Mix the creamed coconut with the boiling water and stir until the coconut is dissolved. Put it to one side to cool a little.

2   Add the tofu and cumin to the nut butter and purée until smooth. Slowly blend in the coconut water.

3   Gently heat the sauce on the hob or in the microwave and pour over cooked vegetables.

Blue Cheese & Yoghurt

A quick and easy dressing to serve with salads and soups. You can make it with any type of blue cheese. It goes really well with crudités, carrot, celery and parsnip dishes. It freezes well.

150g/5½oz Roquefort or other blue cheese
400ml/14fl oz natural unsweetened yoghurt
or fromage frais

Put the cheese and yoghurt into a blender and whiz until you have a smooth mixture. Store in the fridge.

Vietnamese Dressing

A light, fresh tasting dressing that you can use with just about any type of salad or vegetable. An authentic dressing uses Vietnamese mint or Laksa leaf. Unless you are able to grown this yourself Laksa leaf is difficult to obtain so this recipe uses a mixture of fresh mint and coriander instead. This dressing freezes well.

SERVES

50ml/2fl oz rice vinegar

50ml/2fl oz Thai fish sauce

2 tsp sugar

125ml/4 fl oz water

2 cloves garlic crushed

Grated zest of 1 lime

Juice of 2 limes

1 red birds eye chilli very finely chopped OR

1 tsp Sambol Oelek or chilli paste

1 tbsp finely chopped coriander

1 tbsp finely fresh mint

2cm/1 in piece ginger finely grated

Put all the ingredients into a jar with a lid and give them a good shake to thoroughly mix them.

Cooked Salad Dressing

With most commercial mayonnaise made from vegetable oils that are in the 'never eat' category, this war time recipe for a salad dressing is quite useful. You can use it just as you would commercial mayonnaise or salad cream. The dressing will keep for 4 – 5 days in a jar in the fridge.

SERVES

1 tbsp plain flour OR cornflour

2 tsp mustard powder

1 tsp sugar

1 free range egg

1 tbsp olive oil or butter

175ml/6fl oz milk

4 tbsp lemon juice

A pinch of cayenne pepper

A pinch of garlic granules (optional)

1   Mix together the flour, mustard powder, cayenne pepper and sugar. If you are using the adding the garlic granules add these also at this stage.

2   Beat the egg and milk together and whisk in the oil. If you are using butter melt it first. Slowly add this to the flour and mustard whisking everything until it is smooth.

3   Pour the mixture into a saucepan and bring it very slowly to the boil over a medium heat. Keep stirring all the time with the whisk to prevent it from sticking as it thickens.

4   Cook for 2 minutes. Leave it to cool and then whisk in the lemon juice. Season to taste with salt and pepper and extra lemon juice.

Basic Red Mole Sauce

No apologies for repeating the recipe for this sauce simply because it is so useful. The sauce freezes really well so it is worth making a batch for the freezer. Omit the garlic if you are making it for the freezer and add it later.

2 tbsp olive oil

1 large red or white onion finely chopped

3 cloves garlic crushed

3 tbsp cocoa powder

1 tsp chilli powder

2 tsp ground cumin

1 tsp smoked paprika

1 tbsp sweet paprika

½ tsp salt

1 tbsp dried oregano

2 x 400g/14oz cans chopped tomatoes

2 red peppers diced finely sliced or diced

1 Heat the olive oil in a large saucepan. Add the onion, garlic and the red pepper and sauté over a medium heat for 5 to 10 minutes. Do not let the onion or garlic brown.

2 In a small bowl mix together the cocoa powder, chilli, cumin, both types of paprika, salt and oregano. Add this to the onion and pepper mixture, stir well and cook, stirring all the time, for a minute or two to bring out the flavour of the spices.

3 Add the canned tomatoes. Give everything a good stir, bring to the boil, turn down the heat and simmer gently for 10 - 15 minutes.

BREAD, BISCUITS, CAKES & MUFFINS

It is interesting to look at old war time recipes for biscuits and cakes and compare them to modern ones. Three things that stand out are the amounts of sugar, fat and egg that the recipes contain. With all of these ingredients rationed, the old recipes contain far less than the modern ones and interestingly, most of the old recipes taste just as good.

Because it is high in resistant starch and contains little or no gluten, many of the following recipes use fine or 'pinhead' oatmeal. You can usually buy this in health food stores but as you will rarely find it in supermarkets the best thing is to make your own using a blender or food processor. Just put 500g/1 lb 2 oz of flaked oatmeal into the blender and process until you have a powder which is 'coarse to fine', not as fine as flour but much finer than the original oatmeal.

As all grains and cereals are to a some degree inflammatory, in an anti-inflammatory diet a useful trick is to include some strongly anti-inflammatory ingredients that reduce their inflammatory potential and balance things out a little. Ground ginger and cinnamon are powerful anti-inflammatory ingredients and both ground and whole nuts, especially Brazil nuts, are a particularly useful addition to 'sweet' cakes and muffins. When making 'savoury' breads and bakes. ground turmeric, chilli powder, garlic granules and dried herbs, even when used in only small amounts, are a useful addition and interestingly they often enhance the flavour of the baked goods.

Brazil Nut & Oatmeal Tiffin

Quick and easy to make this recipe uses lightly toasted Brazil nuts and fine oatmeal instead of digestive biscuits,

MAKES 16

175g/6oz flaked oats	3 tbsp cocoa powder
125g/4½oz Brazil nuts	3 heaped tbsp dark unrefined sugar
85g/3oz butter	4 tbsp water
4 heaped tbsp raisins soaked for	1 tsp vanilla extract
½ hour in hot water	75g/2¾ oz 70% or 85% chocolate

You will need a 20cm/8 in square tin to make this. Pre heat the oven to 180°C/ 350°F/Gas 4.

1. Put the flaked oats and Brazil nuts into a food processor or blender and process until they form a smooth fairly fine powder. Put them onto a baking tray and bake them for 5 minutes. Take them out of the oven and give them a good stir. Put them back into the oven and cook for another 5 minutes. They should look lightly toasted. Put them to one side while you prepare the rest of the ingredients.

2. Put the butter, water, cocoa powder and sugar into a medium size saucepan and gently heat it until the butter is melted. Keep stirring it over a low heat and cook it for 3 – 4 minutes. This will take the raw taste out of the cocoa.

3. Stir in the vanilla extract and raisins, then add the baked oatmeal and Brazil nuts. Mix thoroughly. The mixture will be quite stiff. Spoon the mixture into the tin and press it down very firmly using the back of a spoon. Cover and leave to cool for at least an hour.

4. Break the chocolate into pieces, put it into a dry bowl and melt it slowly over a saucepan of simmering water. Pour the chocolate over the biscuit base and leave it to set before cutting the tiffin into 16 pieces. Store in an airtight container for up to a week.

Chocolate, Pear & Almond Muffins

This will make 12 large muffins or if you use a cake tin a 20cm/8 in cake.

Makes 12 muffins
350g/12oz peeled, cored and
grated pear
70g/2½oz ground almonds
30g/1oz flaked almonds
3 tbsp dark unrefined Muscavado
sugar
1 tsp baking powder
1 tsp bicarbonate of soda

120g/4¼ oz wholegrain spelt
40g/1½ oz cocoa powder
3 tbsp olive oil
1 large free range egg

Pre heat the oven to 180°C/ 350°F/Gas 4 and grease or line 12 large muffin tins.

1   Mix together the spelt, baking powder, bicarbonate of soda, ground and flaked almonds and cocoa powder.

2   Whisk the oil into the egg and mix this into the grated pear.

3   Add the dry ingredients to the grated pear and egg and mix well. Spoon into muffin tins and bake for 20 minutes.

Chocolate Crunch Biscuits

This recipe is a war time recipe that uses no egg and very little sugar and fat. The biscuits are very easy to make and taste surprisingly good.

Make about 16
2 heaped tbsp unrefined dark
Muscavado sugar
2 tbsp cocoa powder
50g/1¾oz butter

3 tbsp water
½ tsp vanilla extract (optional)
150g/5½oz flaked oatmeal

You will need a 20cm/8 in square tin, preferably silicon bakeware, .

Pre heat the oven to 160ºC/ 325ºF/Gas 3. If the baking tin you are using is metal grease the bottom of the tin really well or line it with baking parchment.

1   Put the butter, sugar, water and cocoa powder into a medium size saucepan and melt the butter over a gentle heat. Stir it well to remove any lumps of sugar and cook, stirring once or twice over a very low heat to 'cook' the cocoa powder and remove the raw cocoa taste.

2   Turn off the heat and add the flaked oatmeal to the butter and cocoa. Mix thoroughly. The mix will be quite dry and become harder to work as it cools. Put it into the prepared tin and using the back of a spoon press it down firmly.

3   Cook for 20 minutes until it is firm to touch. Take it out of the oven and put to one side to cool a little.

4   When it is cool enough to handle put the biscuit onto a chopping board and use a sharp knife to cut it into 16 pieces.

Date & Muesli Bars

Moist chewy biscuits that are quick and easy to make and keep for up to a week in an airtight tin. The mashed banana works wonders as it takes the place of egg and binds the ingredients together.

Makes 9 - 16

2 large ripe bananas

1 heaped tbsp dark unrefined Muscavado sugar

2 tbsp olive oil

120g/4¼ oz chopped dates

30g/1oz pumpkin seeds

3 tsp mixed spice

½ tsp ground ginger

200g/7oz flaked oatmeal

50g/1¾oz chopped pecan nuts or walnuts

You will need a 20cm/8 in greased square tin, preferably silicon bakeware. Pre heat the oven to 160°C/ 325°F/Gas 3.

1. Put the bananas into a bowl and use a hand blender to whiz them into a smooth purée. Add the olive oil and blend until mixed.

2. Mix together the flaked oatmeal, muscavado sugar, mixed spice and ground ginger in a separate bowl. If the sugar is lumpy break it up with your fingers.

3. Stir in the nuts, pumpkin seeds and chopped dates.

4. Add the banana and oil to the oatmeal, seeds and nuts and mix thoroughly. The mixture will be fairly dry. Put it into the prepared tin and, using the back of a spoon, press it down firmly.

5. Cook for 30 minutes until the biscuit is firm to the touch and beginning to look slightly golden around the edge. Take it out of the oven and put to one side to cool a little.

6. When it is cool enough to handle put the biscuit onto a chopping board and use a sharp knife to cut it into 9 or16 pieces.

Rough Oatcakes & Variations

Traditional oatcakes are made from fine oatmeal, salt, some form of fat or oil and water. The oatmeal makes them a 'healthy' biscuit that provides plenty of resistant starch. By adding additional ingredients you can transform these simple biscuits into something quite special. A few variations are included but try experimenting yourself.

Makes a lot

200g/7oz fine oatmeal

100g/3½oz flaked oatmeal

½ tsp salt

Small hand full of sunflower seeds (optional)

Crushed black pepper to taste

4 tbsp olive oil

About 150ml/5 fl oz (¼ pt) boiling water

Line 2 large baking trays with baking parchment or non stick foil.

Pre heat the oven to 180°C/ 350°F/Gas 4.

1 Mix together the oatmeal, salt, pepper and if you are using them the sunflower seeds.

2 Make a well in the centre and pour in the oil and the boiling water and mix until you have a firm dough. If the mixture looks too wet add some more fine oatmeal.

3 Cover the dough and leave it to rest for 10 – 15 minutes.

4 Lightly dust a sheet of baking parchment or a piece of cling film with some fine oatmeal. Put the dough on top and use your hand to flatten it slightly. Sprinkle on some more oatmeal and cover with another piece of baking parchment or cling film. Roll the dough out until the dough is 3 - 4 mm thick.

5 Take off the top piece of baking parchment or cling film and use a 5cm/2 in pastry cutter to cut out the biscuits. Put them onto the baking trays. Re work the pieces of biscuit dough left over into a

ball and repeat the process.

6   Bake for 10 minutes. Take the oatcakes out of the oven and turn them over. Put them back in and cook for another 10 minutes. Leave the oatcakes to cool for a few minutes before putting them onto a wire tray.

Variations

Before adding the oil and water:-

- Add 1 tsp sweet paprika, ½ tsp chilli powder, ½ tsp garlic granules and 1 tsp dried oregano.

- Add 1 tsp smoked garlic granules and 1 tsp ground dried rosemary

- Add 50g/1¾oz basil pesto

- Add 2 tbsp finely grated parmesan and 2 tbsp finely chopped spring onions.

Savoury Oatmeal Biscuits

A chunky savoury oatmeal biscuit that is a variation of classic oatcakes. This recipe uses mild chilli and oregano but rosemary and finely grated parmesan cheese or a tablespoon of basil pesto also work well.

Makes 24

50g/1¾oz fine oatmeal
150g/5½oz flaked oatmeal
50g/1¾oz sunflower seeds
30g/1oz toasted sesame seeds
½ tsp baking powder
2 tsp dried oregano
4 tsp mild chilli powder

1 tsp cayenne pepper
1 tsp garlic granules
4 tbsp olive oil
4 tbsp water
1 large free range egg

Line a large baking tray with baking parchment or non stick foil.

Pre heat the oven to 160°C/ 325°F/Gas 3

1. Mix together the dry ingredients.

2. Put the egg, water and olive oil into a bowl and use a hand blender to mix it together until it is light and fluffy.

3. Add the egg and oil mixture to the dry ingredients and mix until you have a firm sticky dough.

4. Take a tablespoon of the dough, roll it into a ball and then flatten the ball out on the baking tray into a fairly thick biscuit. The dough should make about 24 biscuits.

5. Bake the biscuits for 20 minutes. Turn them over and bake for another 5 minutes.

Digestive Biscuits

Another frugal war time recipe. The original recipe used whole meal flour but this recipe uses wholegrain spelt instead. If you want to make the biscuits into chocolate digestives spread some melted 70% solids chocolate over them when they are cooked.

Makes a lot

175g/6oz wholegrain spelt	1 tbsp sugar OR 1 tsp stevia
60g/2¼oz fine oatmeal	1 tsp baking powder
85g/3oz butter	1tsp bicarbonate of soda
½ tsp salt	50ml/2fl oz milk

Pre heat the oven to 180°C/ 350°F/Gas 4 and line 2 baking trays with baking parchment or non stick foil.

1   Mix together the spelt, oatmeal, salt, sugar or stevia, baking powder and bicarbonate of soda.

2   Rub in the butter until the mixture resembles fine bread crumbs.

3   Add the milk and work the mixture into a soft dough.

4   Lightly dust a sheet of baking parchment or a piece of cling film with spelt. Put the dough on top and use you hand to flatten it slightly. Sprinkle on some more spelt and cover with another piece of baking parchment or cling film and roll the dough out until the dough is 3 - 4 mm thick.

5   Take off the top piece of cling film and use a 5cm/2 in pastry cutter to cut out the biscuits. Put them onto the baking trays. Re work the pieces of biscuit dough left over into a ball and repeat the process.

6   Bake for 10 – 12 minutes until the biscuits are light golden around the edges. Leave to cool for a few minutes before putting them onto a wire tray.

Olive & Anchovy Bites

With the anchovies and cayenne pepper these melt in the mouth biscuits are a healthy non inflammatory treat. They store very well and can be kept in an airtight container in the fridge for up to 2 weeks. You can also freeze them for up to 3 months.

Makes a 40 – 45

175g/6oz whole grain spelt

1 tsp cayenne pepper

50g/1¾oz butter

4 tbsp finely grated parmesan

50g/1¾oz tin anchovy fillets in olive oil roughly chopped

50g/1¾oz chopped salted black olives

1   Place all of the ingredients except the black olives into a food processor and pulse until the mixture forms a firm dough.

2   Put the dough onto a piece of baking parchment and knead in the chopped olives. Wrap the dough in cling film and chill for half an hour.

3   Pre heat the oven to 200°C/ 400°F/Gas 5 and line 2 large baking trays with baking parchment or non stick foil.

4   Put the dough onto a sheet of lightly floured baking parchment or cling film. Cover with another sheet of baking parchment or cling film and roll it until it is 3 – 4 mm thick.

5   Cut it into strips 5cm/2 in wide. Then cut each strip diagonally in alternative directions to make triangles.

6   Put the biscuits onto the baking trays and bake for 8 – 10 minutes until they are golden brown. Cool on a wire rack.

Banana Blue Berry Muffins

You can use fresh or frozen fruit to make these. Use blue berries or black currents. The recipe makes 12 50ml/2 fl oz muffins.

Makes 12

125g/4½oz wholegrain spelt
100g/3½oz ground almonds
1 large free range egg
3 tbsp olive oil
1 heaped tbsp dark unrefined
Muscavado sugar

2 bananas weighing about 300g/10½oz
1 tsp baking powder
1tsp bicarbonate of soda
85g/3oz blue berries or black currents
1 tbsp demerera sugar (optional)

Pre heat the oven to 180°C/ 350°F/Gas 4 and grease the muffin tins.

1   Mix together the spelt, ground almonds, sugar, baking powder and bicarbonate of soda. You may need to break up the lumps in the sugar with your fingers.

2   Put the bananas, egg and oil into a bowl and whiz it with a hand blender until you have a smooth cream.

3   Add the dry ingredients and mix well. Fold in the blue berries or black currents and spoon into the muffin tins. If you are using it, sprinkle the demerera sugar on top and bake for 20 minutes.

Onion & Walnut Muffins

Onions in a muffin? Well yes, and interestingly they do not have a strong onion taste. These savoury muffins are great for breakfast and they also go really well with soup. You can use walnuts or pecan nuts to make them. The muffins taste good and the onions and nuts make them a special anti-inflammatory treat. If you are avoiding wheat use a mixture of fine oatmeal and buckwheat instead of the spelt. These muffins freeze well so make twice the quantity and put some into the freezer.

Makes 8 large muffins or 12 small ones

125g/4½oz white onion roughly chopped

4 tbsp olive oil

1 large free range egg

1 tsp cayenne pepper

1 tsp garlic granules

1 tsp baking powder

150g/5½oz finely chopped pecan nuts or walnuts

175g/6oz wholegrain spelt

Pre heat the oven to 220°C/ 450°F/Gas 6 and grease your muffin tins.

1   Put the walnuts into a blender or food processor and process until they are finely chopped.

2   Put the ground walnuts into a bowl with the spelt and baking powder and mix well.

3   Put the chopped onion with the olive oil, egg, cayenne pepper and garlic granules into a food processor or blender and whiz until you have a smooth purée.

4   Add the onion and egg purée to the walnut and spelt and mix thoroughly. Spoon into muffin tins and bake for 5 minutes then turn the oven down to 200°C/ 400°F/Gas 5 and cook for another 15 minutes.

Oven Dried Tomato & Olive Muffins

Use oven dried tomatoes or sun dried tomatoes. If you are not keen on goats cheese use Brie or Camembert instead.

Makes 8 – 12

225g/8oz whole grain spelt

2 tsp baking powder

½ tsp cayenne pepper

1 tsp garlic granules

3 tbsp finely grated parmesan

100g/3½oz goats log cut into small pieces

3 tbsp olive oil

50g/1¾oz salted black olives with their stones removed

100g/3½oz chopped oven dried tomatoes

1 tbsp chopped basil leaves

1 large free range egg

250ml/9 fl oz milk

Pre heat the oven to 220°C/ 450°F/Gas 6 and grease the muffin tins.

1 Whisk the egg with the milk.

2 Mix together the spelt, cayenne pepper, garlic granules, baking powder and 2 tbsp of the parmesan.

3 Chop the black olives and add them with the chopped tomatoes and chopped goats cheese to the dry ingredients.

4 Stir in the egg and milk and the basil leaves. Mix well and spoon the mixture into the muffin tins.

5 Sprinkle the remaining spoonful of grated parmesan on top of the muffins and bake for 10 minutes. Turn the oven down to 180°C/ 350°F/Gas 4 and cook for another 10 minutes. The muffins should be soft and springy to the touch when they are cooked.

Carrot & Almond Cake

The two main ingredients in this cake are carrots and almonds. The recipe contains quite a lot of sugar as this gives the top of the cake it's characteristic macaroon texture. Unfortunately the sugar puts the cake into the 'naughty but nice' category, only to be eaten once in a while. You can use stevia or another artificial sweetener instead of the sugar but the cake will not have quite the same texture. You can cook this either as a single cake or as muffins.

SERVES 6 – 8

4 large free range eggs separated

Finely grated zest of a lemon

150g/6 oz caster sugar

30g/1oz buckwheat or rice flour

250g/9oz finely grated carrots

250g/9oz finely ground whole almonds

½ tsp almond essence (optional)

3 tbsp pine kernels

Pre heat the oven to 180°C/ 350°F/Gas 4 and either grease and line a 20cm/8 in cake tin or prepare a dozen muffin tins.

1   Grind the almonds in a food processor or blender. Put them into a bowl an mix them with the grated carrots, the lemon zest and the buckwheat or rice flour.

2   Put the egg whites into a large dry bowl and whisk them until they form soft peaks. Whisk in the sugar and if you are using it the almond essence. The mixture will become thick and glossy.

3   Quickly whisk in the egg yolks. Don't over beat or the egg whites will lose their volume. Add about one third of the whisked eggs to the carrots and almonds and mix until the carrots and almonds have loosened. Then gently fold in the rest of the whisked eggs.

4   Spoon the mixture into the prepared cake tin or divide it between the muffin tins. Sprinkle on the pine nuts.

5   Bake the muffins for 20 minutes and the cake for 45 minutes.

Courgette Tea Bread

A strange combination. The courgettes give the loaf a soft moist texture. If you can find them use yellow courgettes. You can use any type of low fat soft cheese. If you are avoiding dairy products use silken tofu instead.

300g/10½oz courgettes grated
1 free range egg beaten
4 tbsp olive oil
4 tbsp unrefined Muscavado
sugar
4 tbsp Ricotta or other low fat soft cheese
175g/6 oz whole grain spelt

55g/2oz fine oatmeal
2 tsp baking powder
1 tsp bicarbonate of soda
1 tsp cinnamon
1 tsp nutmeg

Pre heat the oven to 160°C/ 325°F/Gas 3 and grease and line a 1Kg/2lb loaf tin.

1   Put the egg, sugar, olive oil and Ricotta into a bowl and mix until smooth.

2   Grate the courgettes and mix them into the egg mixture.

3   In a separate bowl combine the spelt, oatmeal, cinnamon, nutmeg, baking powder and bicarbonate of soda.

4   Gradually stir the dry ingredients into the egg mixture until you have a heavy batter. If the mixture looks too thick add a tablespoon or two of cold water. Pour into the prepared loaf tin and bake for 60 minutes. A skewer will come out clean when the cake is cooked.

Chocolate & Hazelnut Polenta Cake

This cake originates from a recipe for a windfall apple cake that was made without eggs. I guess this was at a time when eggs were rationed or hard to come by. The basic cake recipe has evolved over the years. This recipe uses flour, polenta and low fat soft cheese.

If you are avoiding dairy products you can use silken tofu instead of the cheese, and if you are avoiding gluten use fine oatmeal instead of the spelt. The texture will not be the same but the cake will taste just as good. The basic cake recipe can be made with different combinations of ingredients. Some variations are listed below. The cake freezes well.

250g/9oz Ricotta, Quark or other soft low fat cheese.
200g/7oz polenta
200g/7oz whole grain spelt
3 tsp baking powder
3 tbsp dark unrefined Muscavado sugar
85g/3oz melted butter

100g/3½oz toasted hazelnuts with their skins removed
85g/3oz dark chocolate chips
150g/5½oz ready to eat prunes roughly chopped
200ml/7 fl oz water
1 tbsp demerera sugar

Pre heat the oven to 160°C/ 325°F/Gas 3 and grease and line a 20cm/8 in cake tin.

1   Melt the butter and leave it on a very low heat while you prepare the rest of the ingredients.

2   Add the water to the cream cheese and blend thoroughly.

3   Put the polenta, spelt, sugar and baking powder into a bowl and mix thoroughly. Roughly chop the hazelnuts and add them to the flour. Stir in the chocolate chops and the prunes.

4   Add the cheese and water and mix well. Then stir in the melted butter. Pour the cake mixture into the prepared tin and sprinkle the demerera sugar on top.

5   Bake for 1½ to 2 hours. If you test the cake with a dry skewer it will come out clean when the cake is cooked. Leave the cake to cool in the tin for half an before turning it out.

Variations

Omit the hazelnuts, prunes and chocolate chips.

The original windfall apple cake was made from 2 - 3 desert apples that were cored and then chopped into small pieces, 50g/1¾oz raisins or sultanas that had been soaked in hot water for an hour and 50g/1¾oz chopped walnuts.

Another variation is to use 150g/5½oz chopped ready to eat apricots and 50g/1¾oz lightly toasted flaked almonds.

Spongy Gingerbread

Another war time recipe that at the time was for a 'luxury' cake. Golden syrup was a rare ingredient. The recipe has been slightly modified to use mashed banana instead of golden syrup. Use buckwheat instead of spelt if you are avoiding gluten.

SERVES 8

200g/7oz wholegrain spelt

85g/3oz fine oatmeal

4 tsp ground ginger

1 tsp mixed spice

3 heaped tbsp dark unrefined Muscavado sugar

1 tsp baking powder

1 tsp bicarbonate of soda

3 tbsp olive oil

50g/1¾oz raisins or sultanas

1 large eating apple

1 large free range egg

2 peeled bananas weighing 200g/7oz

6 tbsp cold water

You will need a 20cm/8 in square tin, preferably silicon bakeware, .

Soak the raisins or sultanas for an hour in warm water or tea.

Pre heat the oven to 160°C/ 325°F/Gas 3. If the baking tin you are using is metal grease the bottom of the tin really well or line it with baking parchment.

1   Mix together the spelt, oatmeal, ground ginger, mixed spice, baking powder and bicarbonate of soda. Add the sugar and rub it well in with your hands to break up any lumps.

2   Put the bananas, egg and olive oil into a bowl and whiz it with a hand blender until you have a smooth creamy purée.

3   Core the apple, grate it and mix it with the drained raisins into the banana purée.

4   Add the purée to the oatmeal, mix well and pour it into the baking tin. Cook for 45 minutes until golden and firm to the touch.

Courgette Crown Bread

Adding grated courgette and cheese can transform an ordinary loaf into something special. Use yellow courgettes if you can get them.

450g/1 lb grated courgette
500g/1lb 2oz whole grain spelt
Sachet fast acting bakers yeast
4 tbsp finely grated parmesan
1 tbsp sesame seeds

½ tsp cayenne pepper
1 tsp garlic granules (optional)
2 tbsp olive oil
Tepid water

You will need a 23cm/9 in round tin to make this. If you are using a metal tin grease it well.

1 Mix the spelt with the yeast, cayenne pepper, parmesan and garlic granules if you are using them.

2 Add the grated courgette and mix it into the flour.

3 Slowly add some tepid water and mix the dough with your hands until you have a firm dough. How much water you need depends on the amount of fluid in the courgettes.

4 Knead the dough on a floured board for about 10 minutes until it is smooth and 'stretchy'. Cover and leave the dough to prove until it has doubled in size.

5 Knead the dough for a couple of minutes and divide it into 8 pieces and roll these into balls. Put one ball in the centre of the baking tin and arrange the others around the outside. Brush with milk or water and sprinkle the sesame seeds over the top. Cover and leave the bread to rise until it has doubled in size.

6 Pre heat the oven to 200°C/ 400°F/Gas 5 and bake the bread for 30 minutes. It is cooked when it sounds hollow when you tap the bottom.

Classic Soda Bread

Traditionally soda bread is made with buttermilk. As buttermilk is difficult to find these days, use a mixture of natural unsweetened yoghurt and water instead. Soda bread made from wholegrain wheat or spelt never rises as well as soda bread made with white flour but it tastes much better and it makes wonderful toast. Any bread made with chemical raising agents needs to go into a very hot oven as soon as the dough is mixed. It should only be kneaded lightly, just long enough to shape it. This is because the raising agent starts working as soon as it comes into contact with fluid, so extended kneading means that you end up with a loaf that does not rise well.

500g/1lb 2oz wholegrain spelt
2 tsp bicarbonate of soda
Hand full of pumpkin seeds
Hand full sunflower seeds

200ml/7 fl oz natural unsweetened yoghurt
200ml/7 fl oz water

You will need a lightly greased baking tray and a 24cm/10in cake tin with a solid base to make this. Putting the cake tin upside down on top of the bread will help it rise.

Pre heat the oven to 220°C/ 450°F/Gas 6.

1   Mix together the spelt, bicarbonate and seeds in a large bowl.

2   Whisk the yoghurt and water together and add this to the flour. Mix well, turn it onto a floured board and quickly shape it into a round.

3   Put the dough onto the baking tray, cover it with the inverted cake tin and and bake it for 30 minutes. Remove the tin, reduce the temperature to 180°C/ 350°F/Gas 4 and bake it for another 10 – 15 minutes. When it is cooked the bread should sound hollow when the base is tapped.

Carrot & Coriander Bread

This is a moist soda bread that keeps well. You can use carrot, butternut squash or sweet potato. Try adding different combinations of herbs and spices as well.

375g/13oz wholegrain spelt
85g/3oz fine oatmeal
40g/1½ oz flaked oatmeal
1 tsp garlic granules
1 tsp cayenne pepper (optional)
1 tsp baking powder
1 tsp bicarbonate of soda
3 tbsp chopped coriander OR
1 tbsp ready made coriander pesto

Hand full pumpkin seeds OR
roughly chopped pistachio nuts
250g/9oz finely grated carrots
300ml/10 fl oz (½pt) natural unsweetened
yoghurt
300ml/10 fl oz (½pt) water

You will need a greased 20cm/8 in square tin to make this.

Pre heat the oven to 200°C/ 400°F/Gas 5

1 Mix together the spelt, fine oatmeal, flaked oats, pumpkin seeds, baking powder, bicarbonate of soda, garlic granules and if you are using it the cayenne pepper.

2 Stir the grated carrot into the dry ingredients.

3 Whisk together the yoghurt, water and chopped coriander or coriander pesto and stir this into the carrot and dry ingredients. Quickly mix to form a soft dough.

4 Spoon the dough into the prepared tin and bake for 20 minutes. Turn the oven down to 180°C/ 350°F/Gas 4 and cook for another 20 minutes. When it is cooked the bread should sound hollow when the base is tapped.

Oatmeal & Spelt Soda Bread

The original recipe for this is a Victorian recipe for a 'healthy' bread made from whole grain flour, oatmeal and butter milk. It's spongy texture is a long way from being anything like 'bread' as we know it but it tastes good, lends itself to many different variations and it is quick and easy to make. It makes an ideal base for pizzas.

100g/3½oz wholegrain spelt
100g/3½oz fine oatmeal
1 tsp baking powder
1 tsp bicarbonate of soda
2 tbsp olive oil

Hand full pumpkin seeds
125ml/4 fl oz natural unsweetened yoghurt
200ml/7 fl oz water

You will need a 24cm/10 in silicon cake tin or spring form tin with a loose base to make this. If you are using an ordinary tin grease it well. Pre heat the oven to 220°C/ 450°F/Gas 6.

1   Mix together the spelt, oatmeal, baking powder and bicarbonate of soda.

2   Whisk together the yoghurt, olive oil and water and add this to the dry ingredients. The mixture is quite runny and it will start bubbling as soon as the yoghurt and water is added to the flour, so mix it quickly to form a batter and pour it into the baking tin.

3   Put it into the oven straight away and bake for 12 - 15 minutes. By this time it should be lightly browned and firm to the touch.

Variations:

•   For a chilli bread add 2 tsp mild chilli powder and 1 tsp oregano,

•   For a herb bread add 1 tsp garlic granules, 1 tsp dried rosemary and 1 tbsp chopped black olives.

•   Adding a tablespoon of pesto makes something really different.

DESSERTS

For most of us the word desserts conjures up images of food that is far from healthy. Can deserts be part of a healthy anti-inflammation diet? Well yes they can, especially if they are preceded by a healthy anti inflammatory first course. Remember, "it's what you do most of the time not what you do some of the time" that really matters so once in a while indulge yourself and do not feel guilty about it.

Hazelnut Nut & Chocolate Roulade.

At first sight this recipe looks difficult but it is actually quite easy to make. The recipe uses chocolate with orange liqueur as a filling. You could also use some raspberries, fresh or frozen, instead of the liqueur.

SERVES 6 – 8

For the roulade

175g/6oz finely ground lightly toasted Hazelnuts

30g/1oz buckwheat flour

4 large free range eggs

2 tbsp caster sugar

Filling

350g/12oz silken tofu OR Ricotta or other low fat soft cheese

125g/4½oz dark chocolate, minimum 70% solids

2 -3 tbsp orange liqueur

Pre heat the oven to 200°C/ 400°F/Gas 5. Line a 32cm (13in) x 23cm (9in) Swiss roll tin with non stick baking parchment or non stick foil.

1   Put the hazelnuts and buckwheat flour into a blender or food processor and process until the hazelnuts are ground to a fine powder.

2   Separate the eggs and put the egg whites into a large, dry bowl. Whisk the egg whites until they form soft peaks. Then whisk in the sugar.

3   Add the egg yolks to the egg whites and quickly whisk them in. Don't over whisk or the mixture will lose its volume. Carefully fold in the ground hazelnuts.

4   Pour the mixture onto the prepared Swiss roll tin and spread it out evenly. Bake in the middle of the oven for 8 – 10 minutes. It should be just firm to the touch and springy when cooked. Take it out of the oven and cover it with a sheet of baking parchment and a clean tea towel. Leave it to cool.

5   To make the filling beat the tofu or soft cheese until it is smooth

and then beat in the orange liqueur.

6   Break the chocolate into a dry bowl and put it over a saucepan of
    gently simmering water to melt. Leave it to cool a little, then beat it
    into the tofu/cheese mixture. Leave it to cool a little before
    assembling the roulade.

7   To assemble the roulade. Take off the tea towel, put a large board
    on top and turn the roulade over. Remove the baking parchment.
    Using a sharp knife, trim off the edges. You need to do this as it
    makes it easier to roll the roulade up.

8   Spread the chocolate mixture evenly over the roulade. Pick up the
    baking parchment along a long side of the roulade and gently roll
    the roulade over using the baking parchment to move it forward.
    Roll the roulade up in the baking parchment and put it into the
    fridge until you are ready to serve it.

Banana Soufflé

Served the moment it comes out of the oven a soufflé is one of the most impressive dishes you can make. The timing is critical but the preparation is straightforward and most of it can be done in advance.

Making a banana soufflé is really easy, more like magic than cooking. The secret is to use egg whites that have been kept in the fridge for a day or two. Unfortunately the recipe uses sugar as it just does not work if you make it with an artificial sweetener. Needless to say this puts it into the 'sometimes' eat category.

You will need 2 large 300ml/10 fl oz ramekin dishes.

SERVES 2

1 large banana mashed	Butter for greasing
1 tsp cornflour	2 egg whites
1 tbsp water	55g/2oz caster sugar plus
squeeze of lemon juice	caster sugar for dusting

Pre heat the oven to 200°C/ 400°F/Gas 5 and put a baking sheet into the oven.

1 Grease 2 large ramekin dishes and dust them with caster sugar. The dusting with caster sugar is important as it helps the soufflé to rise.

2 Mix the cornflour with the water to make a thick paste add this to the mashed banana. Blend thoroughly until you have a smooth purée.

3 Put the egg whites into a large, clean, dry bowl and whisk them until they start to form peaks. Add a small squeeze of lemon juice and continue whisking until the egg whites are really thick and silky and forms peaks. Slowly whisk in the sugar.

4 Mix a third of the egg whites into the banana purée, then gently fold in the rest of the egg white.

5   Fill the ramekins with the soufflé mixture and smooth the top to make a flat surface. Run your thumb around the top edge of the ramekin. This prevents the soufflé from sticking and it helps it to rise evenly.

6   Take the baking tray out of the oven, put the ramekins onto it and bake for 15 minutes. Serve immediately.

Cranachan

A traditional Scottish dessert made from toasted oatmeal. The oatmeal is soaked overnight in whisky and honey and then mixed with soft cheese and raspberries. Most recipes you see today do not soak the oatmeal and they use whipped cream instead of the cheese. This recipe uses half fromage frais and half thick Greek yoghurt instead of the cream but you could also use a soft low fat soft cheese like Ricotta or Quark. The whisky gives the desert it's characteristic flavour. Whether you use Whiskey and how much you use is a matter of personal taste.

SERVES 4

300ml/10 fl oz (½pt) fromage frais

300ml/10 fl oz (½pt) thick unsweetened Greek yoghurt

85g/3 oz flaked oats that have been toasted golden brown

3 tbsp Whisky

3 tbsp runny honey

450g/1lb raspberries

Toasted flaked almonds to garnish

1   Mix 2 tbsp of the honey and 2 tbsp of the whiskey with the toasted oatmeal and leave it to soak.. How long you soak it for is a matter of taste. The longer it soaks the softer it becomes.

2   Beat the fromage frais and yoghurt together until they are thoroughly blended and then stir in the remaining honey and whisky.

3   Crush half of the raspberries lightly with a fork and stir them into the yoghurt mixture.

4   Put a layer of whole raspberries into the bottom of 4 desert glasses. Put in a layer of the yoghurt mixture and then a layer of the oatmeal. Continue until you have used all the raspberries. Finish with a layer of yoghurt. Garnish with the toasted flaked almonds before serving.

Chocolate Brownies

Use any type of nut to make these, almonds, pecan nuts, hazelnuts and walnuts all work. You can serve the brownies on their own or with fromage frais. You will need a 20cm/8 in square cake tin.

Makes 12 – 16

100g/3½oz nuts

100g/3½oz butter

100g/3½oz 70% or 85% chocolate

2 large free range eggs beaten

40g/1½ oz wholegrain spelt

40g/1½ oz polenta

3 tbsp dark unrefined Muscavado sugar

2 tsp baking powder

Pre heat the oven to 180°C/ 350°F/Gas 4 and grease and line the cake tin.

1. Roughly chop the nuts and toast them for 4 minutes. Take them out and give them a stir, put them back in and toast them for another 4 minutes. Take them out of the oven and put them to one side while you prepare other ingredients.

2. Turn the oven down to 160°C/ 325°F/Gas 3.

3. Break the chocolate into a dry bowl, add the butter and sugar and put the bowl over a saucepan of gently simmering water until the chocolate and butter have melted. Stir until the mixture is smooth. Turn off the heat.

4. Put the spelt, polenta, baking powder and nuts into a bowl. Add the melted chocolate and the beaten eggs and mix well. Spoon into the prepared tin, smooth over the surface and bake for 25 - 30 minutes. The brownies will feel slightly springy in the middle when they are cooked.

Leave to cool before cutting into 12 or 16 pieces.

Russian Raspberry Pudding

A simple very easy recipe that can be eaten hot or cold. Fresh raspberries are best but you can also use frozen raspberries. The recipe uses a small amount of sugar. You can substitute Stevia or another artificial sweetener if you wish. When it is hot, straight from the oven, this recipe smells delicious and I think it is the best way to eat raspberries.

SERVES 4

450g/1lb raspberries

2 tbsp caster sugar.

150ml/5 fl oz (¼ pt) fromage frais

150ml/5 fl oz (¼ pt) thick unsweetened Greek yoghurt

2 large free range eggs

1 tbsp flour

1 tbsp Demerera sugar

Pre heat the oven to 150°C/ 300°F/Gas 2

1   Put the raspberries into a greased gratin dish and sprinkle then with 1 tbsp of caster sugar. Put the dish into the middle of the oven and leave them to heat through for 10 minutes.

2   Beat the fromage frais, yoghurt, eggs, flour and remaining tbsp caster sugar together. Pour this over the raspberries and sprinkle on the demerera sugar. Put the raspberries back into the oven on the top shelf. Leave the oven on the same temperature.

3   Cook for about 45 minutes until the top is light golden brown and firm to touch

Strawberry & Lemon Cheesecake

A cooked cheesecake that you can make with either a low fat soft cheese or silken tofu. The base is made from an over sized chocolate crunch biscuit. Don't be put off by the length of the recipe. It is actually quite easy to make. The cheesecake does not freeze but it will keep in the fridge for up to 2 days.

SERVES 6 – 8

For the base
2 heaped tbsp unrefined dark
Muscavado sugar
2 tbsp cocoa powder
50g/1¾oz butter
3 tbsp water
½ tsp vanilla extract (optional)
150g/5½oz flaked oatmeal

For the cheesecake
500g/1 lb Ricotta, Quark or other low fat
soft cheese
50g/1¾oz caster sugar

150ml/5 fl oz unsweetened Greek style
yoghurt
3 large free range eggs separated
Juice and zest of a lemon
½ tsp vanilla extract
500g/1lb 2oz strawberries or other soft fruit

You will need a 24cm/10 in silicon cake tin or a spring form tin with a loose base to make this.

Pre heat the oven to 160ºC/ 325ºF/Gas 3. If the baking tin you are using is metal grease the bottom of the tin really well or line it with baking parchment.

1   Put the butter, sugar, water and cocoa powder into a medium size saucepan and melt the butter over a gentle heat. Stir it well to remove any lumps of sugar and cook, stirring once or twice over a very low heat to 'cook' the cocoa powder and remove the raw cocoa taste.

2   Turn off the heat and add the flaked oatmeal to the butter and cocoa. Mix thoroughly. The mix will be quite dry and become harder to work as it cools. Put it into the prepared tin and press it down VERY firmly.

3   .Cook for 20 minutes until it is firm to touch. Take it out of the oven and put to one side to cool a little while you make the cheesecake. Turn the oven down to 150°C/ 300°F/Gas 2.

4   Put the Ricotta, and yoghurt into a bowl and beat until smooth. Add the vanilla extract, lemon zest, lemon juice and egg yolks and mix well.

5   Put the egg whites into a large dry bowl and whisk until they form soft peaks. Beat in the caster sugar.

6   Fold a third of the egg whites to the cheese mixture. Gently fold in the remaining egg whites.

7   Take the cooked base out of the tin and remove the baking paper from its base. If you are using a metal tin grease the sides and the base. Put the cooked base back into the tin.

8   Pour in the cheesecake mixture and bake in the middle of the oven for 1½ hours or until a skewer comes out clean when you put it into the centre of the cheesecake.

9   Turn off the oven and leave the cheesecake to cool in the oven with the door open. The top may have cracked but don't worry about this. Remove from the tin and chill for 2 – 3 hours before arranging the strawberries or mixed fruit on the top.

Avocado & Pistachio Semifreddo

Avocados are packed full of healthy Omega-3 oils. In some parts of the world they are eaten as a dessert. Their rich texture makes them perfect for a smooth creamy ice cream or semifreddo. This recipe uses yoghurt but you can use pouring cream instead. Adding rice flour or cornflour to the yoghurt prevents the yoghurt from splitting as you heat it.

SERVES 4 – 6

300ml/10 fl oz (½pt) unsweetened
natural yoghurt
1 tbsp rice flour
3 large free range eggs
3 tbsp caster sugar OR stevia to taste

2 ripe avocados
Zest of 1 lime
Juice of ½ lime
30g/1oz pistachios roughly chopped

1   Put the yoghurt into a bowl with the rice flour and and sugar and whisk until you have a smooth mixture. Whisk in the eggs one at a time.

2   Pour the yoghurt and egg mixture into a saucepan and bring it very slowly to the boil over a medium heat, gently whisking to prevent it sticking. Turn the heat down and cook for 4 - 5 minutes until the mixture thickens. Cover and leave to cool. Stir occasionally to prevent a skin forming.

3   Remove the stones from the avocados and scoop the flesh into a bowl. Add the lime zest and lime juice and use a hand blender to process the avocado until It is smooth and creamy.

4   When the yoghurt and egg mixture is cool stir it into the avocado. Mix thoroughly and then stir in the pistachios. Pour into a 500ml/18fl oz container, cover and freeze for at least 6 hours. Serve cut into slices.

Chocolate & Hazelnut Parfait

A really delicious desert that is made from home made chocolate and hazelnut spread and yoghurt. It will keep in the freezer for up to 6 months. Use an ice cream maker if you have one. Alternatively you use 125ml/4 fl oz size silicon muffin tins to make individual parfaits.

MAKES 6 individual parfait or a
700ml/25 fl oz/1¼pt tub
200g/7oz hazelnuts
3 tbsp cocoa powder
1 tsp vanilla extract
3 heaped tbsp dark unrefined
Muscavado sugar

50g/1¾oz butter
2 tbsp water + 6 tbsp water
300ml/10 fl oz (½pt) natural
unsweetened yoghurt

Pre heat the oven to 180ºC/ 350ºF/Gas 4

1   Put the hazelnuts onto a baking tray and roast them for precisely 8 minutes. Take them out of the oven, put them onto a damp tea towel and rub them. Most of the skins will come off, don't worry about any that are left on.

2   Put 2 tbsp water, the butter, the cocoa powder and the sugar into a small saucepan and gently heat it until the butter is melted. Keep stirring it over a low heat and cook it for 3 – 4 minutes. This will take the raw taste out of the cocoa. Stir in 1 tsp vanilla extract and leave the mixture to cool slightly.

3   Process the hazelnuts in a food processor or blender until they release their oil and form a smooth paste. This will take between 5 and 10 minutes.

4   Pour the chocolate mixture into the hazelnuts and process until everything is thoroughly mixed. Slowly add 6 tbsp cold water, 1 tbsp at a time until you have a smooth slightly runny paste.

5   Add the yoghurt and process until you have a smooth mixture.

6   Spoon the parfait into individual containers and freeze until solid. Alternatively process using an ice cream maker.

Chocolate & Raspberry Fromage Frais
This is probably one of the quickest and easiest deserts you can make.

SERVES 4

120g/5 oz dark chocolate

150g/5 oz raspberries, fresh or frozen

2 tsp finely grated zest of a lemon

300g/10½oz fromage frais

1   Break the chocolate into pieces and put it into a small dry bowl. Put the bowl on top of a saucepan of gently simmering water and leave it to melt slowly.

2   Take the bowl off of the saucepan, stir in the lemon zest and leave the chocolate to cool for 15 minutes.

3   Stir the fromage frais into the chocolate and then gently stir in the raspberries. Spoon it into glasses. Chill well before serving.

Ginger Chocolate Cheesecake

A cheesecake with a difference. It tastes good but the crystallised ginger and sugar put it firmly into the 'sometimes eat' category. The cheesecake freezes well.

SERVES 6 – 8

350g/12oz silken tofu

200g/7oz mascarpone or other cream cheese

125g/4½oz 70% chocolate

50g/1¾oz butter

3 large free range eggs

100g/3½oz crystallised ginger finely sliced

2 tbsp unrefined dark sugar

1 heaped tsp ground ginger

1 – 2 tbsp spiced rum (optional)

For the base

2 heaped tbsp unrefined dark Muscavado sugar

50g/1¾oz butter

2 tbsp water

3 - 4 tsp ground ginger

½ tsp grated nutmeg

150g/5½oz flaked oatmeal

You will need a 20cm/8 in tin, preferable silicon bakeware, which is at least 3 cm deep to make this.

Pre heat the oven to 160°C/ 325°F/Gas 3. If the baking tin you are using is metal line the base with baking parchment.

1   First make the base. Mix together the flaked oatmeal, ground ginger and nutmeg.

2   Put the butter, sugar and water into a small saucepan and melt the butter over a gentle heat. Stir it well to remove any lumps of sugar.

3   Pour the melted butter and sugar into the flaked oatmeal and mix thoroughly. The mix will be quite dry and become harder to work as it cools. Put it into the prepared tin and press it down firmly.

4   Cook for 20 minutes until the base is firm to touch. Take the base out of the oven and put to one side. Turn the oven down to 150°C/

300°F/Gas 2.

5 Put the tofu, mascapone, eggs, sugar, ground ginger and, if you are using it, the spiced rum, into a bowl and mix thoroughly with a hand blender.

6 Break the chocolate up and put it into a dry bowl with the butter. Put this over a saucepan of water that is simmering very gently. Slowly melt the chocolate and butter. Leave it to cool for 5 – 10 minutes.

7 Stir the melted chocolate and butter into the tofu, cheese and egg mixture and then gently stir in the sliced crystallised ginger.

8 If you are using a metal baking tin grease the sides of the tin above the base. Pour the cheesecake mixture onto the base and cook for 1 hour. Turn off the oven and leave the cheesecake inside the oven with the door slightly open to cool before putting into the fridge. Leave the cheesecake for at least 3 hours before serving.

Apricot Clafoutis

You can make this recipe with more or less any type of fresh soft fruit. Apricots and plums work well and if can get hold of cherries and damsons when they are in season they are really good. Use an artificial sweetener if you prefer not to use sugar. The egg whites that are not used in the recipe can be stored in the fridge for a couple of days and used in other recipes. They can also be frozen.

SERVES 6

500g/1lb 2oz apricots	4 large free range eggs
1 tbsp apricot kernels (optional)	2 egg yolks
3 tbsp flour	300ml/10 fl oz (½pt) milk
3 tbsp caster sugar or more to taste	300ml/10 fl oz (½pt) unsweetened Greek yoghurt

Grease a shallow baking or gratin dish and sprinkle the inside with some sugar. This will help prevent the clafoutis from sticking.

Pre heat the oven to 180°C/ 350°F/Gas 4.

1 Cut the apricots in half and remove the stones Lay the apricot halves on the dish. The apricot kernels inside the stones give this an intense almond like taste so break open some of the stones with a nut cracker and remove a tablespoon of the kernels.

2 Mix together the flour and the sugar and whisk in the whole eggs and egg yolks.

3 Whisk the milk and yoghurt together and slowly add it to the egg and flour mixture. You should have a smooth custard. Stir in the apricot kernels.

4 Pour the batter over the apricots and bake for 30 to 40 minutes until the custard is golden and rise. Serve hot or cold.

RECIPE INDEX

9 781999 624859